cellulite SOLUTION

A Doctor's Program for

Losing Lumps, Bumps,

Dimples, and Stretch Marks

◆

HOWARD MURAD, M.D.

 ST. MARTIN'S GRIFFIN ❧ NEW YORK

www.stmartins.com

Design by Patrice Sheridan

LIBRARY OF CONGRESS CATALOGING-IN-PUBLICATION DATA

Murad, Howard.
    The cellulite solution : a doctor's program for losing lumps, bumps, dimples, and stretch marks / Howard Murad.
        p. cm.
    Includes an index (p. 221).
    ISBN 0-312-33461-3 (hc)
    ISBN 0-312-33462-1 (pbk)
    EAN 978-0-312-33462-8
    1. Cellulite. 2. Women—Health and hygiene. 3. Skin—Care and hygiene.
4. Reducing diets. 5. Reducing exercises. I. Title.

RA778.M955 2005
613.7'045—dc22

                                                                2004051466

10   9   8   7   6   5   4   3   2

Note to the Reader

The information contained in this book is not a substitute for the advice of a qualified medical professional, who should always be consulted before beginning any new health, diet, or exercise program. If you are pregnant, nursing, or taking any kind of prescription medications, or if you are under the special care of a physician, be sure to have your doctor's advice and supervision. Your physician should be aware of all medical conditions you have as well as the medications and vitamin supplements you are taking. He or she should be the authority on optimum dosage requirements for all nutrients and vitamins.

Contents

The Cellulite Solution

Introduction

Cottage cheese skin? Orange peel thighs? You probably picked up this book because you see these problems every day. You are not alone. Lumpy, textured skin affects 90 percent of women who have gone through puberty. Women just like you, who have tried everything to smooth their bodies—from leg lifts and fad diets to high-priced creams and "miracle" tablets—only to come away with, at best, minor, temporary results and a lighter wallet. In fact, most people, including many in the medical profession, have resigned themselves to the thought that there is no way to treat cellulite and stretch marks permanently.

I have some great news for you. Cellulite and stretch marks are no longer an inevitable fact of life. With some modifications to your nutritional habits and lifestyle, you can experience the first scientifically proven method of smoothing cellulite. Implementing the steps I outline in this book will provide your body with a complete, healthy environment and all of the tools it needs to repair uneven, lumpy skin on its own.

Have You Had Enough of Those Tried and Tired Cellulite Remedies?

Many popular theories say that cellulite is the result of excess fat in the body, and therefore dieting is the answer. Others say that cellulite is caused by an overabundance of water, and therefore dehydration of the affected areas is the answer. Well, the popular theories on cellulite and stretch marks are wrong. Have you ever gone on a successful exercise or dieting program only to find that you lost excess weight but the cellulite was still there? Have you ever attempted to parch the offending areas of your thighs or backside using topical caffeine or some other dehydrating agent only to find the area plumped up again as soon as you drank some water? You are not alone.

The conventional theories are partially correct. The problem does involve fat. It does involve water. But the solution is not as simple as removing the excess fat and water from your body. As you probably know, there are many thin women with cellulite, and there are many fully hydrated women without it. What is important is not the amount of fat or water in your body, but how we treat the fat and water that are there.

In practicing dermatology in Los Angeles for the past thirty years, I have treated thousands of women, from working moms to famous actresses. Regardless of their age or body type, their most frequent concerns are cellulite and stretch marks. I know very well how troubling these conditions can be for women. Unfortunately, there has been no available treatment with scientifically proven results—until now.

The Water Principle Primer

Using the experience and knowledge gained through years working in the fields of science and medicine, I developed a revolutionary theory that has become known as the *water principle*. It is the basis for my breakthrough program. As we age, our bodies lose the ability to utilize water as they did when we were younger. Over time, our cells and the other areas of our bodies that need hydration break down and become unable to hold onto water, leaving them weakened and less effective. This water that your cells can no longer utilize now passes right through you or, even worse, stays in between the tissues of your body, swelling your ankles or puffing your eyelids. I call this wasted water, and to attain smooth skin, you need to put it back in your cells where it will keep you firm and supple.

When your cells are not fully hydrated, they cannot function at their optimal level. This leads to much of the tissue damage that we call aging. For example, dehydrated skin is more likely to weaken and succumb to all sorts of ravages that lead to cellulite and other problems. This dehydration and deterioration of cells can be due to a simple dietary deficiency of vital cell-hydrating nutrients.

By taking the necessary supplements every day and making a few changes to your diet, you can reverse the breakdown of your skin and prevent future damage. I have been using a combination of cell-repairing nutrients such as pomegranate extract and essential fatty acids for years, with amazing results. I had proved in numerous studies that applying the water principle to my patients' treatments did wonders for their wrinkles. I wondered if it could be as effective in the treatment of cellulite and stretch marks, and I resolved to find out. I began by studying the anatomy of cellulite and questioning the common theories and treatments that have not worked.

My first question was, Why does cellulite have a bumpy texture while ordinary fat does not? Although the popular theories on cellulite state that it is ordinary fat and we need to treat it as such, it was clear to me that this was not the case. Ordinary fat's function in the body is to create a soft, frictionless padding for the muscles, organs, and skeletal system. Because of this, it is smooth, shapeless, and able to glide effortlessly over the tissue it surrounds. This is not the case with cellulite and stretch marks. They are rigid and have a definite shape.

My second question was, Why is the fat that makes up cellulite visible while ordinary fat is not? The fat that makes up cellulite is clearly different from ordinary fat. I knew that traditional methods of treating cellulite as normal fat were not effective, and I soon discovered why. The standard cellulite treatments can't possibly work because they are treating the wrong problem. Throughout this book you will learn the answers to these questions and what you can finally do to treat cellulite in a way that actually works.

My next step was to gather a research team to test my theories in comparison to the traditional methods of cellulite treatment. We investigated how cellulite fat cells differ from normal fat cells and tested my theories on treating them as such. The results were smooth thighs and big smiles on my patients' faces. In fact, in a double-blind, randomized, placebo-controlled study performed by an independent laboratory, the test subjects experienced a 78 percent increase in skin firmness after eight weeks of taking the nutrients I discuss in this book!

Finally there is a program that offers you the first definitive road map to reducing dimpling and improving stretch marks that is actually backed by science. Cellulite is not a new problem. What is new is the solution. At long last, we are ready to tackle this last beauty taboo head-on. After years of exhaustive research, I can say without question that the method I have designed works.

A New Kind of Treatment

This is the answer to women's most common beauty afflictions, one that doesn't involve pricey creams, invasive surgery, or multiple high-tech treatments. In fact, many of the vital components of this method are available in your local supermarket or health food store. Many cellulite treatments on the market are solely topical, you rub them on your skin. The right topical ingredients can do wonders for your ridges and dimples. However, the benefits are limited because cellulite is deposited below the surface of the skin where topical creams cannot always reach. The core philosophy of my method is to create a complete environment for healthy tissues within your body. You can achieve this with a three-part program: (1) internal nutrients, (2) application of a topical cream to nourish your surface skin, and (3) some minor lifestyle adjustments. When you take care of your teeth, you don't only brush; you floss and visit the dentist too, each step working synergistically with the others to give you optimal oral health. It is the same with treating cellulite. Nutritional supplements and minor dietary changes are major forces in resolving both cellulite and stretch marks, and they can improve your skin's firmness at the same time. To be effective, we need a comprehensive approach to healthy skin that works not only on the epidermis, the skin's outer layer, but also on the dermal layer below the skin's surface. Most of us think of skin care as restricted to topical applications, but my philosophy is to effect change from the inside as well as from the outside. I call this *internal skincare,* and it is the only way to completely heal your skin.

With the current worldwide obsession to have the perfect body, people are now more conscious of every imperfection. Since women are working out more and looking after their bodies at a furious pace, cellulite and stretch marks are more of a concern than ever. Women understandably feel self-conscious about their bodies, as they are constantly under scrutiny by men as well as other women, and especially by their own highly critical eyes. Far too many women never show their legs, wear a skirt, or go to the beach because they are embarrassed by dimpling and stretch marks.

Contrary to popular opinion, cellulite is not the result of too much fat in your body. The actual cause of cellulite is water damage and weakening of the skin cells and connective tissue. Cellulite is caused by skin that has deteriorated to the point that buoyant fat cells are able to push into the dermis, the middle layer of skin, and show through the surface. By simply adding key skin-hydrating, cell-fortifying nutrients such as glucosamine, essential fatty acids, amino acids, lecithin, and antioxidants to your diet, you can repair, rehydrate, and revitalize your skin, forcing stubborn fat cells back invisibly below the surface—and keeping them there. These nutrients work in conjunction with topical agents that hydrate, firm, and stimulate blood flow, leaving you with tightened, supple, smooth skin that you will be proud to show off.

◆

The Three Keys to a Smoother You
Repair
Rehydrate
Revitalize

Necessary Nutrients for Smooth Skin

The way to get rid of cellulite and stretch marks and keep them from coming back is simply a matter of nutrition—nutrition for your body's cells and connective tissue. I have always said, "Before there was medicine, there was food." Long before penicillin, doctors and medicine men prescribed foods that contained the specific nutrients their patients needed in order to heal and prevent illness and tissue damage. Instead of addressing only the symptoms of cellulite and stretch marks, my program confronts the causes. It gives your body the nutrients it needs to repair weakened skin tissue, thereby diminishing the damage that leads to cellulite. If you eat the right foods and nutrients, you can keep your cells and connective tissue well nourished, hydrated, and vital. This is the most important step in firming your tissues and pushing that pesky fat back where it belongs—below the visible layer of your skin.

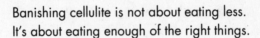

Banishing cellulite is not about eating less.
It's about eating enough of the right things.

These healthy, skin-fortifying ingredients are easy to find in grocery stores, natural food stores, and vitamin shops. They are safe and effective, and don't come with designer price tags. Add these essential nutrients to your diet in the form of food and supplements, in addition to some easy, do-it-yourself topical treatments and simple lifestyle alterations, and you will have smooth skin again in no time. This book features a complete guide to the necessary nutrients and how they work to prevent and repair cellulite. If you can't wait to jump into the program, you can move on to Chapter 6.

PATIENT TESTIMONIAL

◆ ◆ ◆

Andrea
Age: 42
Occupation: Massage therapist
Areas of concern: Thighs and stomach

Personal testimony: As a massage therapist, I am very aware of my body and I also feel quite knowledgeable about vitamins and products for the skin. I am probably the most skeptical person also, because I've had clients tell me about cellulite creams they use and other methods they've tried to get rid of it. When I started the study, I went to the gym regularly and felt I was in good shape. Then due to changes in my work schedule, I stopped working out. I was very surprised to notice a visible improvement in my stomach and thighs, and my skin felt tighter, even though I wasn't doing any exercise. But something else happened too. I usually need a heavy painkiller every day during my period, but since I started taking these vitamins I don't need them anymore. I've also noticed that I feel calmer during stressful times; my blood pressure dropped from 130/90 to 120/90. Whatever is happening, I love it and I am motivated to keep doing it. It's so easy to just take a few pills and apply the gel.

Clinical Program
- daily intake of supplements to address cellulite as outlined in this book
- topical application of cellulite serum

Clinical Results
Initial visit: stage-3 cellulite
Final visit: stage-1 ½ cellulite

Additional Clinical Observations
Water measurements:
Visit 1 Intracellular <u>19.0</u> Extracellular (noncompartmentalized) <u>16.1</u>
Visit 2 Intracellular <u>19.1</u> Extracellular (noncompartmentalized) <u>16.9</u>
Final Intracellular <u>20.2</u> Extracellular (noncompartmentalized) <u>15.9</u>

% Body Fat
Visit 1: 46.3
Final visit: 42.6 (a decrease of 3.7%)

BMR (Basal Metabolic Rate, number of calories used at rest)
Visit 1: 1,414
Final visit: 1,511 (an increase of 97 calories burned per day at rest)

◆

The cell is immortal. It is merely the fluid in which it floats that degenerates. Renew this fluid at regular intervals, give the cells what they require for nutrition, and as far as we know, the pulsation of life can go on forever.
> —Dr. Alexis Carrel,
> Winner of the Nobel Prize in Medicine

◆

One

The Anatomy of Cellulite and Stretch Marks: Causes and Effects

You know that fatty tissue is found in most parts of your body to varying degrees. It primarily functions as a protective cushion for your organs and as an energy reserve. When you reduce your normal intake of food, your body automatically burns its own reservoir of stored fat. On a low-calorie diet, fat comes off in many areas, but the cellulite bulges remain.

The fat beneath the skin that you see in the diagram on page 13 is the fat that covers your muscles. It is the fat that accumulates when you eat more calories than you use, and the fat that comes off when you diet and exercise. This fat does not contribute to cellulite or stretch marks. When you lose weight, no matter what diet-exercise program you use, the percentage of body fat decreases, but there is no measurable loss of cellulite. This is because the body cannot utilize fat trapped in the dermal layer, the fat that actually contributes to cellulite, as fuel. The main problem with most other cellulite treatments is that they address only the fat below the skin and fascia. This approach can't work because the subdermal fat cannot react to treatment as the normal fat can. Unfortunately, that dermal fat that causes cellulite is there to stay. The good news is that with a few simple steps every day, you will never have to notice it.

The Skin's Layers

The stratum corneum is the uppermost layer of skin. It is made up of dead and dying cells held together by a lipid (fat) membrane. As these cells fall off, new cells are produced at the bottom of the epidermis, pushing everything above them up. Think of the stratum corneum as the roof of your house. It is the protective shield against the ravages of the environment.

Living epidermis is the top layer of skin, encompassing the stratum corneum and the skin cell layer below it. It contains dying cells that have less and less water as they move up into the stratum corneum. This is an important defense against incoming damage such as the sun's rays and other environmental stresses.

The dermis is made up of fibrous material, collectively known as the body's matrix, plus other elements. In a way it is a microcosm of the rest of your body. It has blood vessels, nerves, connective tissue, glands, and other organelles such as hair follicles. The dermis makes up the bulk of your skin. It gives the skin its resiliency. A healthy dermis shows up as firm skin; an unhealthy dermis shows up as wrinkles and sags. The dermis is made of

- substances called glycosaminoglycans (or GAGs), semi-solid material that has a great deal of water-bonding ability.
- collagen and elastin, the "frames" of the dermis. If you think of the dermis as a mud hut, the matrix would be the

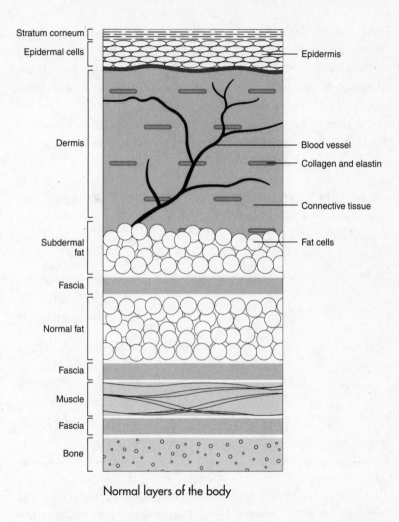

Normal layers of the body

mud, and collagen and elastin would be the straw fibers holding it together. The breakdown of collagen and elastin is the direct cause of wrinkles.

Subdermal fat is the fat that is trapped below the dermal layer where it cannot be burned as fuel. If the dermis and epidermis above it become damaged and weaken, this fat will push its way toward the surface and become visible cellulite.

Fascia is fibrous material that separates various body components. If you think of a steak, the fascia is the dense white material that separates the meat from the fat.

Normal fat appears when we overeat, and it is burned as fuel when we exercise. It does not contribute to cellulite.

PROS AND CONS OF DIET AND EXERCISE

Method	It Does	It Doesn't
Weight loss diet	reduce fat	reduce dimpling, because cellulite is formed by fat that cannot be metabolized
Exercise	build up muscle, reduce fat	reduce dimpling, because cellulite fat deposits are trapped in pockets where they cannot be readily used as fuel

While weight training, stretching and toning exercises, and aerobics are good for your body, they will not cure cellulite because they target only fat and muscle, not the dermal layer where cellulite lives.

SEPARATING CELLULITE FROM NORMAL FAT

Cellulite	Normal Fat
affects women only	affects women and men
concentrated primarily at the inner, outer, and posterior thighs; inner knees; upper and lower abdomen; hips; buttocks; lower back; back of upper arms; ankles	occurs everywhere on the body
when squeezed, appears to have ridges, lumps, irregularities	when squeezed, is smooth in texture
within the skin	below the skin
cannot be used as an energy source by the body	can be accessed by the body as an energy source

The Cellulite Time Line

Cellulite was first mentioned by European physicians at the turn of the nineteenth century. In the medical literature, it has been referred to by a wide variety of ominous-sounding names, including mesenchymal disease, cellulitic dermo-hypodermosis, and panniculosis.

In 1920, the French scientists Alquier and Paviot first described the condition.

In 1966, the Spanish dermatologist M. Bassas Grau confirmed that fluid accumulates around cellulite tissue.

In 1972, Doctors G. Muller and F. Nurnberger showed that where cellulite occurs there is also a decrease in the quantity of elastin fibers in the dermis and a rearrangement of the collagen bundles.

In 1994, Professor Sergio Curri, an Italian anatomopathologist and molecular biologist, gave cellulite its scientific validation by carrying out studies comparing cellulite to normal fat and thereby establishing cellulite as a specific syndrome. Despite this, specialists more often than not still treat cellulite as though it were normal fat when prescribing treatments. This is why past cellulite treatments have shown few to no visible results.

Causes of Cellulite

Cellulite is caused primarily by hormones. In fact, the reason men never get cellulite is likely that they have much less estrogen in their bodies than women do. Another factor is genetics. If your mother had cellulite, you are more likely to have it too. These hormonal and hereditary factors allow the dermis to become damaged more easily in specific areas. Dermal fat cells in cellulite areas are closer to the surface because the dermis has been damaged. This tissue in women tends to be less flexible than in men, which is another reason that it is more easily ruptured by age and the environment. For some reason, women tend to bruise on their thighs very easily and have spider veins. This implies weakend blood vessels, one of the primary causes of cellulite. This may be hormonal, or genetic, but it is evidently true.

As the dermis sustains this damage, it loses water and weakens. Eventually, it breaks down so much that the dermal fat that had been resting discreetly below it begins to push its way conspicuously into it. If the epidermis also becomes weakened and dehydrated, it thins, and the cellulite becomes visible from the surface. To get rid of cellulite and stretch marks, we need to focus on repairing the dermis and the epidermis, not on burning fat.

Definitions of cellulite and recommendations for how to treat it have been a controversial subject for decades. Most often, cellulite is described as a cosmetic problem, which it is. However, cellulite is also a medical condition.

Cellulite can be defined as a medical disorder first observed as microscopic changes within the skin, which are not apparent on the surface. These invisible changes, however, manifest themselves as cosmetic problems later on, which is what we commonly associate with dimples. Cellulite is a progressive condition. It may start out as a minor imperfection, but it can become a major stumbling block to self-esteem and a healthy body.

The Two Types of Body Tissue

As I came to understand the body in a broad way, I realized that there are truly only two types of tissue.

- **Cells**. Though skin cells are not the same as, say, liver cells, their basic traits are the same. All cells have a membrane or protective wall comprised of lipids, or fats, and lecithin. Within this cell wall is a substance called cytoplasm, and within the cytoplasm is the cell's nucleus. The nucleus is the control center, or brain, of the cell. Both the cytoplasm and the nucleus are predominately made up of water.

   The heart, brain, bones, and epidermis are made up of cells.
- **Connective tissue**. This tissue has very few cells and is predominately made up of fibrous material. It connects the various organs to the rest of the body. Connective tis-

sue contains the body's matrix (glycosaminoglycans, or GAGs). This is a semisolid matter made of materials such as hyaluronic acid, a water-loving substance that can actually attract up to 1,000 times its weight in water. The building block for hyaluronic acid is glucosamine. Collagen and elastin keep the connective tissue firm and hold its shape. The building blocks for collagen and elastin are the amino acids in the foods we eat.

Blood vessels, nerves, tendons and ligaments, and dermis are connective tissue.

To repair cellulite, we need to strengthen and hydrate the cells and connective tissue in your body by feeding them with the nutrients and water they need to stay healthy.

Blood Vessels

The primary factor that contributes to cellulite is interference with your blood vessels' ability to circulate nutrients. As the skin is the outermost part of your body, nutrients need to travel all the way through the blood vessels to reach it. As the blood vessels are the connective tissue of the heart, they can be damaged in much the same way as the skin's dermis—and with the same destructive results.

Damaged blood vessels do not have the reach that healthy blood vessels do. Women with cellulite frequently have damaged capillaries (spider veins) and varicose veins, and are prone to bruising and discoloration. Anything that strengthens the vessels and improves blood flow to the area also strengthens the dermis and the skin cells above it. Repaired blood vessels once again are able to bring the necessary nutrients and water to the dermis and epidermis to further repair the cell walls and connective tissue. This reduces dimpling as well as broken capillaries and varicose veins.

◆

Cellulite is not a static condition. If left untreated, cellulite can and does get worse. The best treatment is early intervention.

Cellulite Exposed

The thigh area is most susceptible to cellulite accumulation. If you look at normal healthy thigh skin, the epidermis on the surface is smooth. The skin is firm because the dermis is thick and undamaged. The bundles of collagen and elastin are strong. Capillaries extend into the uppermost regions of the dermis, providing a blood supply of nutrients and clearing fluids.

Ultrasound scans of normal thigh tissue show dense, hydrated tissue with little wasted water. With a microscope, we can see the activity of fibroblasts. These are cells within connective tissue that produce collagen and elastin. If you think of a fibroblast as an apple tree, collagen and elastin would be the apples. In a healthy thigh, the fibroblasts are actively producing these firming frames within your dermis. The fat cells in the dermis are not swelling or clumping together. They are quite distinct and of normal diameter. Most important, there are no cellulite fat deposits showing through the skin.

Now let's compare that to an unhealthy thigh. As a result of damage to the blood vessels, you may see some damaged capillaries or spiderlike varicose veins on the skin's surface. The stratum corneum, the outermost layer of the skin, is dry and rough to the touch. You may see some flaking of the skin, which is caused by dehydrated surface skin cells breaking off. The skin is loose and sags due to damaged connective tissue that has lost its ability to keep the skin firm. The dermal fat cells within the unhealthy thigh are beginning to swell, and fibrous bands are starting to form around them. Finally, and probably most troubling of all to women concerned with the appearance of their skin, there likely are patches of cellulite. The dehydrated and undernourished dermis and epidermis are too weak in certain areas to keep the dermal fat in check.

This is why traditional methods such as weight loss cannot possibly work. Cellulite is not a "fat" problem—it is a "dermal" and "cellular" problem. Therefore, methods need to be directed toward modifying the adjacent connective tissue and skin cells rather than the fat cells.

The Reason for Cellulite's Texture

Fat cells are surrounded by fibrous bands called septa. As the cells are damaged, these bands harden and become rigid. With the progression of cellulite, the weakening dermis loses its ability to hold the fat cells in place. This newfound freedom of motion allows the fat to push its way into the dermis. The primary function of the dermis is to make connective tissue, so as the fat cells push their way into the dermis, even more septa (which is made of—you guessed it—connective tissue) form around the fat, making them even more rigid as they move toward the skin's surface.

The hardening septa are no longer elastic enough to expand with the fat cells. The fat begins to squeeze out the sides of the fibrous material much like a balloon that is blown up with a rubber band wrapped around it. This is why cellulite has a rough, bumpy texture while ordinary fat is smooth and frictionless. The longer

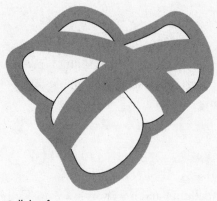

Cellulite fat

the condition progresses, the harder the septa become, accounting for the later stages of cellulite, in which it is more rigid.

Key Components of Cellulite
blood vessel disruption
damage to the dermis
"wasted water" buildup
fat cells swelling and moving closer to the surface
thinning epidermis

Dimple Detection

There are two basic types of cellulite: soft and solid.

Soft cellulite slides easily over the underlying tissue and tends to occupy large areas. It shakes with bodily movement and is much more noticeable than solid cellulite.

Solid cellulite is thick tissue that clings strongly to underlying tissues. It is generally found on young women in good physical condition. Solid cellulite is often sensitive to the touch.

How Advanced Is Your Cellulite?

Press or squeeze the tissues between your thumb and index finger or between your palms. If cellulite is present, the skin ripples. At a more advanced stage, the ripples are noticeable without applying any pressure.

The Stages of Cellulite

You may have cellulite and not even know it. Cellulite starts out deep in the dermal layer where you can't see it.

Stage 1

The earliest events in the formation of cellulite are invisible because they occur at the dermal level. Deterioration of the dermis is the first stage of cellulite formation. Blood vessels in the affected areas begin to break down, which causes a loss of capillary networks in the dermis. As they continue to deteriorate, the skin can no longer receive all of the nutrients it needs, causing even further degradation of the dermis and epidermis. Water begins to seep out of the damaged blood vessels and collects between the tissues as wasted water. Fat cells begin to swell to two or three times their original size and start clumping together. At this stage, the epidermis is still healthy, and the dermis is relatively healthy. There are not yet visible manifestations of cellulite.

Wasted water is also beginning to accumulate in stage-1 cellulite. In my research center, I study patients with various ailments such as acne, wrinkles, and cellulite. I do several tests, checking, among other things, their blood pressure, lean tissue percentage, and intracellular and extracellular water levels. I can often tell when a patient has early, not-yet-visible cellulite by doing a bioelectrical impedance analysis. A very small electric current is run through a person's body. Depending on how fluidly the current travels, the apparatus can tell how much wasted water is impeding its flow. If I find an excess of wasted water, odds are that precellulite tissue breakdown has begun.

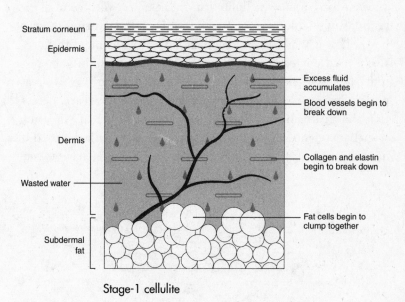

Stage-1 cellulite

Stage 2

In the second stage, the deterioration of the dermis is advanced. Some regions may have normal blood flow while adjacent regions have markedly reduced blood flow. Fat cells become even more swollen and begin pushing out and upward against the ever frailer dermis. This exacerbates the blood flow problem as well, because the blood vessels are pushed aside by swelling fat deposits. This prevents nutrients from reaching the skin, weakening it further. This cycle of tissue breakdown hastens the

development of cellulite. Often in this stage, wasted water that
has been wandering aimlessly through the body accumulates to a
larger degree in the affected areas. The surface effects are still
minimal, yet the "orange peel" look of the skin can be detected
with a pinch test. In general, surface lumpiness or unevenness is
visible at this stage.

You can see how cellulite can sneak up on you from all di-
rections with a number of attacks on the various tissues in your
body. That is why I recommend an inclusive treatment that creates a total environment of health and vitality within your system. Inclusive health implies emotional self-care as well as
physical care. You may also be beginning to see how early detec-
tion and treatment may prevent cellulite altogether. If you catch
it early enough, and begin to supply your skin with the food it
needs to remain firm and youthful, you may never have to see

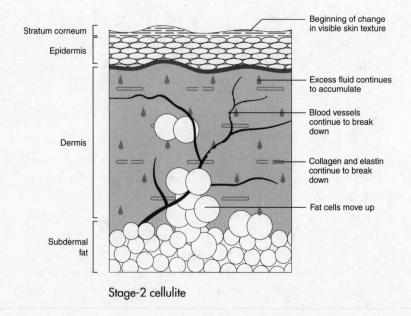

Stage-2 cellulite

these imperfections. Not to mention the wealth of benefits that these nutrients give to your internal organs and connective tissue that you can't see but are sure to feel.

Stage 3

This stage is a continuation of the processes observed in stage 2. The deterioration of the blood vessels has begun to affect the metabolism of the skin's tissues. Loss of nutrients from the blood vessels reduces the body's ability to create proteins and repair itself, which can lead to thinning of the dermis. The hard deposits called septa begin to form around fat cells in the skin. By stage 3, the orange peel effect is visible even without pinching the skin, and the cellulite begins to take on a rough, bumpy feel.

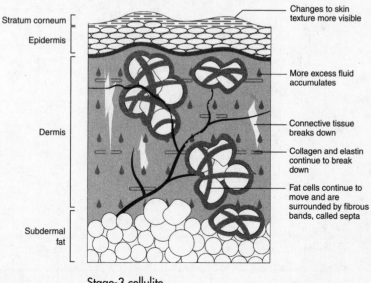

Stage-3 cellulite

Stage 4

In this final stage of cellulite, you can easily see lumps in the dermal region: clumps of fat surrounded by hard protein layers. You can also feel hard nodules by pinching the skin in afflicted regions. Severe cellulite usually has been present for a number of years by the time stage 4 is reached. At this stage, cellulite is accompanied by a lack of firmness due to an advanced deterioration of the skin, both in the surface and dermal layers. This stage of cellulite can be painful, especially after standing for long periods of time when fluid retention in the legs is at its peak.

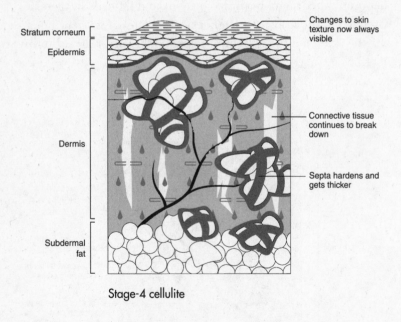

Stratum corneum

Epidermis

Dermis

Subdermal fat

Changes to skin texture now always visible

Connective tissue continues to break down

Septa hardens and gets thicker

Stage-4 cellulite

Cellulite not only is a cosmetic problem, it can also be painful in its most advanced stages.

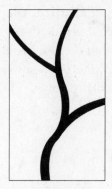
Healthy blood vessel

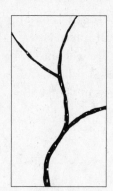
Damaged blood vessel

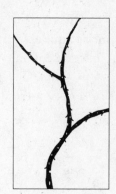
Extensively damaged blood vessel

CELLULITE STAGES

1	blood vessels begin to deteriorate, especially in the upper dermis	fluid accumulates outside of the cells— "wasted" water	changes are not visible
2	dermis deteriorates further	blood vessels become pushed aside as fat cells swell and move toward the surface	minimal orange peel texture visible when pinched
3	beginning of damage to collagen and elastin synthesis	fibrous bands (septa) begin to surround fat cells	significant orange peel texture visible by pinching
4	hard nodules can be felt	pain and tenderness	always visible

The earlier you begin treating your cellulite, the more success you will have. However, even if you don't begin treatment until you are well into stage 4, don't despair. With my program, all degrees of cellulite can be improved because we are repairing the damage in your body that actually causes cellulite.

Some Wisdom About Stretch Marks

Although the title of this book is *The Cellulite Solution,"* I often refer to cellulite and stretch marks together. This is because they have many similarities. Stretch marks are also caused by damage to the dermis. They are simply a more acute version. In the case of stretch marks, the damage is focused in areas of your body that were specifically stressed for a long period of time. The greatest similarity between cellulite and stretch marks is that they are both evidence of damage to the dermis, the elastic middle layer that gives skin its shape.

Think of a rubber band that is stretched out over time. It loses its elasticity and becomes weak. The same thing happens with your connective tissue. As parts of it become damaged and brittle, their newly ridged texture and lack of elasticity become visible.

Stretch marks occur when the dermis is constantly stretched with growth, weight fluctuations, pregnancies, and various diseases. As this happens, the skin loses elasticity and the connective fibers break, which show through the surface as rippled formations.

Resulting inflammation may then cause damage to the melanocytes, the cells in the skin that give it its color. Depending on your natural skin coloring, stretch marks begin as raised pink or reddish to dark brown marks that later turn a brighter purple. This color may be due to damage to the blood vessels as the tissue is stretched. Gradually the marks flatten and fade to a color that is a few shades lighter than your natural skin tone. Over time, this lack of pigment results in the white or translucent scars associated with mature stretch marks.

DIFFERENCES BETWEEN CELLULITE AND STRETCH MARKS

Cellulite	Stretch Marks
A complex disease or problem that starts with damage to the vascular system. Its causes are both hormonal and genetic.	Caused by acute damage to specific areas of the body that are stretched.
Affects 80–90% of women; rarely seen in men.	Affects 70% of adolescent females, 40% of young males, 90% of pregnant women (during the sixth and seventh months of pregnancy).
Most common on thighs, hips, buttocks, knees, upper arms, abdomen.	Most common on abdomen, thighs, breasts in women; armpits in men.
Can affect any woman.	Affects adolescents experiencing growth spurts, bodybuilders who practice strenuous and repetitive exercise, users of topical and systemic steroids, people with massive weight gain and loss (including pregnancy), and people with certain diseases such as tuberculosis.

Two

◆

The Water Principle:
The Source of All Vitality

◆

Fact: Without water, there is no life as we know it.
Fact: As we age or have disease, we lose water in our
tissues.
Fact: Anything that is not living has no water.
Conclusion: The common pathway to all aging and
disease is water loss.

In order to understand how to effectively address cellulite and
stretch marks, it is necessary to understand the core principle behind my breakthrough treatment. The water principle is the theory I developed that enables people to utilize water in the most
efficient way to give their body the optimal level of health and vitality so it can repair conditions such as cellulite and stretch marks.

Drinking enough water is only the beginning. With age and

disease, our tissues become less capable of utilizing the water we drink. In short, the water principle is a comprehensive approach that repairs our tissues so they are again capable of utilizing this water.

The Water Principle: The Fountain of Youth

How to Repair Cells and Connective Tissue to Prevent Water Loss

You know that water is essential for life. You have heard the common wisdom that you need to drink eight glasses of water a day. There is no question that you need to provide your body with enough hydration to make up for what it expends in breathing, sweating, and general daily function. However, it is even more important to ensure that your body uses this water efficiently and effectively, that it doesn't go to waste.

What happens when you drink eight glasses of water a day? Chances are that you are in the bathroom eight times a day as well. All of that water that you are trying to replenish your body with is just passing right through you. This is because as we age, our body's cells break down and lose the ability to hold onto water. A baby's body is 75 percent water. By the time we reach middle age, our body's water content can be as low as 50 percent. Anything that is no longer living has no water. A damaged cell that cannot maintain its water is like a pocket with a hole in it. You can keep putting money in it, but it doesn't do you any good because it just passes right through. But once you repair your cells, they will hold onto all of their needed water, and prevent a number of age-related ailments.

Independent studies as well as studies in my own lab have shown the benefits of attracting water to the tissues. I often put patients on the water principle program. In addition to the benefits to their specific ailment, such as acne, wrinkles, or cellulite, there consistently is a decrease in body fat, an increase in skin and muscle tone and firmness and, of course, increased cellular hydration.

Your Body's Chest of Drawers

Your body contains two kinds of compartments that house and utilize its water: cells and connective tissue. Cells make up your muscles and organs, including your surface skin. Connective tissue is the fibrous material that binds your muscles and organs in place, and connects one organ to another. Unfortunately, as we age and are exposed to environmental damage, our cells and connective tissue break down. They lose the ability to attract and hold onto all of the water they need in order to function at their optimal levels, like they do in a baby's body. The water that seeps out wanders aimlessly through the spaces between cells and connective tissue. This is noncompartmentalized or "wasted" water.

This water is not only useless, it causes problems. It builds up in inconvenient areas, leaving you with puffy ankles or eyelids. This water should be inside the cells and connective tissue throughout your body, keeping your heart, lungs, brain, liver, and skin healthy and vital, but it isn't. Your body can be full of this water and still be dehydrated, because the water is dangling just out of reach, unavailable to the areas that need it. My water principle program focuses on healing your cells and connective tissue and enabling them to become and remain fully hydrated and vital—to take back and use that wasted water for the health and well-being of your entire body. Throughout this book you will learn how a body-hydrating program is the only way to reduce cellulite.

Look at a baby's skin. It is firm, vibrant, and elastic. Now look at your skin. What do you notice? The tone may be unbalanced. It is not as firm. It may be wrinkling. It is dryer and more brittle. These are the visible effects of the difference between optimal and less than optimal connective tissue and cellular water levels.

A baby's cells are at the strongest point that they will be in his or her life. They have solid cell walls that can lock in all of the body's water and therefore function at their highest level. This is true for the cells all over the baby's body, including brain cells, liver cells, and heart cells. However, as skin is the body's most visible organ, it is easiest to see the effect of this optimal hydration by looking at the skin.

Since the molecular structure of water is the essence of life, the man who can control that structure in cellular systems will change the world.

—Dr. Alber Szent-Gyorgy, winner of the Nobel Prize in Physics

---

People frequently ask me what is happening to their skin as they age. I often use the analogy of a tennis ball. Think of a brand-new tennis ball as a cell in a baby's body. It is strong and buoyant. When you hit it, it bounces high and functions at its highest level. Now think of a ball that you have been using for a while. It is not as firm as a new ball. When you squeeze it, it gives. It doesn't bounce as high as it used to. The reason is that with use and damage inflicted on the ball, it has developed tiny holes in its outer shell, enabling the air inside to escape. And while there is air all around it, the ball has no way of attracting and utilizing this air, so it now functions at a lower level.

The cells in our body are very similar. As we age, our bodies are subject to countless environmental insults, such as stress, pollution, sunlight, the foods we eat, and many more. Although the causes may be different, the results are the same. Our cell walls become damaged, allowing the precious water that keeps them functioning slowly to escape. Maybe we are drinking a lot of water. But it often becomes wasted water throughout our body, all around our cells but not inside them. The cells are incapable of attracting and retaining water as they did when we were younger.

The second compartment is the connective tissue, which in the skin is the dermis. It can be compared to a sponge. If a sponge does not contain any water, it is dry and brittle. It is inflexible and can break apart. If a sponge is full of water, it is thicker, flexible, and more elastic. The same applies to the body's connective tissue. If connective tissue stays well hydrated and full of essential nutrients, it is strong, elastic, and youthful. If it does not get these nutrients, it succumbs to environmental damage. The connective tissue weakens and loses its ability to hold onto water. Eventually it breaks down, causing conditions such as cellulite, stretch marks, and wrinkles. An older person's skin's connective tissue is dry and damaged, much like a dehydrated sponge. It bruises with the slightest injury in the same way that the sponge tears with the slightest force. If we rehydrate these tissues, they are far less susceptible to tearing and bruising.

To increase the water-holding properties of a sponge, we would need to increase the material it is made of. It is the same with the body's connective tissue. As we increase the matrix by providing the body with its building blocks, glucosamine and amino acids, it is able to hold onto more water, making it firmer, smoother, and more resilient.

As skin is a visible organ, looking at it provides a window into your cellular and connective tissue health throughout your body. Do you have visible cellulite and stretch marks? Is your skin wrinkling? Is it displaying a loss of elasticity? When you pinch the skin on your hand, does it wait a beat before returning to its normal shape? Is your skin dry? If you can see any of these signs of aging and damage, chances are that your other organs are in a similarly weakened state.

Can anything be done about this water loss? Absolutely. While it is true that natural, or intrinsic, aging is inevitable, the environmental aging that is the result of such problems as pollution, sun damage, cigarette smoke, and internal stresses can be reduced or prevented, and the damage caused to our cells and connective tissue can be reversed. What follows is a guide to repairing your cell walls in a way that is proved to reduce cellulite and stretch marks and to allow every part of your body, from your brain to your skin, to be youthful, healthy, and vibrant.

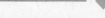

Compartments of Water
1. Cells
2. Connective tissue
3. Noncompartmentalized—wasted water

Life is defined by water. Aging and disease is defined by water loss.

A Simple Triple-Tier Program

The cellulite prescription I detail in the upcoming chapters is a three-pronged approach. Internally, it involves strengthening and healing the cell walls to maintain water levels and functionality, and strengthening and healing the connective tissue. Externally, it involves the use of topical agents to soothe and strengthen the stratum corneum (the outer layer of the skin). This will protect the skin from environmental damage and thereby prevent the resulting loss of water and nutrients. Finally, the program involves some simple lifestyle changes that I address in Chapter 7. If you follow this program, the cells and connective tissue throughout your body will benefit enormously. You will be healthier, less susceptible to premature aging, and have firmer skin and connective tissue all over. First I focus on the skin, to show how my water principle can repair your cellulite and stretch marks.

To reduce cellulite and stretch marks, we must do three things: (1) repair cell damage, (2) repair connective tissue damage, and (3) repair the stratum corneum.

Repair Cell Damage

What we need to do to keep the water inside our cells is repair the cell walls. Our body is like a factory, and it is a truly remarkable one at that. It is constantly repairing damage done to its cells and connective tissue. However, the body often lacks the raw materials necessary to make these repairs. Like a factory, with age the body often needs more and more raw materials to do the same work.

Remember my tennis ball example. If you wanted to prevent the air from continuing to escape from it, you could take it to a factory that would put a layer of rubber around it. But what if the factory didn't have any rubber? You would need to provide

Healthy cell

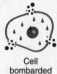

Cell
bombarded
by free
radicals and
inflammation

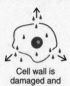

Cell wall is
damaged and
water seeps out

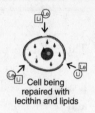

Cell being
repaired with
lecithin and lipids

that too. Once the factory has the rubber it needs, it can take it from there and make any necessary repairs.

The same is true for your body. It knows how to heal your cells. That is one of its primary functions. The problem is that you probably don't get enough of the ingredients in your diet necessary to repair cell walls. Your cell walls are made up of lecithin and lipids, among other things. Because lecithin is found in egg yolk, for example, I often tell my patients who do not have high cholesterol to include whole eggs as part of their diet.

Lipids or fats are another component of cell walls. Prime examples are essential fatty acids. They are "essential" because they are necessary for maintaining a healthy body, yet our bodies are unable to produce them. Other lipids can be produced, but as we age we produce less of them so we need to supplement them in our diet. The problem is that we eat "bad fats" and not enough of the good fats, so our body uses these bad fats to help repair the cell membranes. These bad fats are more subject to damage by free radicals and inflammation, thereby making the problem worse.

In order to get your body to rebuild its damaged cell walls, you need to supply it with the necessary ingredients. Then it will do the rest. Essential fatty acids are found in cold-water fish, as well as some nuts, seeds, and vegetable oils. You can also take supplements that contain these ingredients, which I discuss in detail throughout the book.

Essential fatty acids do more than just build up cell walls. They actually have the ability to extract wasted water from between your cells, where it does no good, and infuse it inside your cells, where it benefits your body. And this water stays inside the cells now that you have reinforced their walls by adding lecithin and lipids to your diet. Not only does this allow all of your body's cells to function as they are supposed to, it also reduces the bloating, swollen ankles, and puffy eyelids that are the result of wasted water buildup. The added benefits are what it does for your cellulite.

Your body is poised to spring into action to repair the damage that time and the environment have done to your cells. It just needs the raw materials to complete this task. A diet rich in lecithin and essential fatty acids will provide your body with the raw materials it needs to rebuild and reinforce your cell walls and keep the water where it belongs—inside your cells.

Repair Connective Tissue Damage

Environmental and internal damage and stresses can break apart connective tissue in the same way that they break apart cell walls. Like your cell walls, connective tissue is made up of substances that our diets rarely provide in sufficient amounts. The skin's connective tissue is the dermis, which is made up of the body's matrix. The dermis contains collagen and elastin, which are made up of amino acids, while the rest of the matrix is made up of GAGs, including, for example, hyaluronic acid. The building block for hyaluronic acid is glucosamine.

A good example of the powerful effects a vital nutrient can have on the body is the treatment of osteoarthritis. This form of arthritis is caused by a weakening of the tendons and ligaments, which are the connective tissue of your body's skeletal system.

Simply providing your body with the glucosamine it needs to repair this weakened tissue can reverse the debilitating pain of arthritis. Glucosamine works on the connective tissue throughout the body, not just in the skeletal system. If your body receives this badly needed nutrient and the ingredients necessary to metabolize it, the brittle, weak connective tissue in your skin becomes as firm and vital as it was years ago, which means you can say good-bye to many of the wrinkles, sags, and dimples that we have all come to accept as part of the "normal" aging process.

Providing your cells and connective tissue with these necessary nutrients will increase the function of all of your organs, from your skin inward. This will be clearly evident when you look at yourself. The patients I put on a diet rich in these nutrients were proved in independent laboratory tests to have a 34 percent reduction in their wrinkles in just five weeks. Sound too good to be true? It gets even better.

Not only will you be healthier and have fewer wrinkles, your cellulite and stretch marks will fade too. After we strengthen and reinforce your cell walls and connective tissue, they will stay firmly in place. They will no longer be pushed aside by the buoyant dermal fat cells that are forcing their way to the surface and creating that annoying dimpling called cellulite. The visible surface of your skin, just like the cells and connective tissue throughout your body, will be firm, smooth, strong, and youthful. And so will you.

Three

◆

Repairing Damage

There are hundreds of theories explaining the causes of aging and damage—from toxins to free radicals to inflammation—and there are likely many causes that haven't even come to light yet. The experts will argue about the causes until you are too confused to know what to do. The important thing is not the cause but the result. No matter what causes aging and damage, the result is the same—loss of water from within your tissues. In Japan they have a saying, "Fix the problem not the blame." Regardless of what causes it, the problem is water loss resulting in weakened tissues and imperfections such as cellulite. This is what we need to fix.

To achieve smooth, dimple-free, healthy skin, we need to repair this damage and replace the lost water. Your first line of defense against cellulite is your connective tissue. The treatments and nutrients that I describe in this section will repair the connective tissue throughout your body. The connective tissues that specifically apply to your cellulite, however, are your blood vessels and your dermis.

Cellulite Stage 1: Blood Vessels

The first stage of cellulite development is blood vessel deterioration. This begins to occur long before the visible signs of cellulite are present. The function of your blood vessels is to transport nutrients, oxygen, and water throughout your body to all of the tissues that need them.

The majority of what we think of as blood is water, with some blood cells and nutrients thrown in the mix. As free radicals, inflammation, and a host of other sources of damage assault your blood vessels, their integrity weakens and tiny holes develop in their walls. At first, these holes are too small to allow your blood cells to escape but not too small to prevent the water from seeping out. This is the water that was being brought to the cells and connective tissues all over your body—in this case your skin cells and your dermis. The water that seeps out of your blood vessels never arrives inside these tissues that need it so desperately. It seeps out and wanders the areas outside of your body's compartments as wasted water, where it not only gives your body no benefit, but is retained, leaving you bloated and swollen.

Eventually, the damage to the blood vessels takes its toll on their functionality. These blood vessels become less and less able to deliver nutrients and oxygen to your hungry skin, especially as they continue to sustain the damage that they are subjected to every day.

Earlier in this book, I compared the body to an automated factory. It is programmed to fix any problems that arise. Our body's ideal state is called homeostasis. This is the condition in which every part of the body, every system that makes it up, is functioning at its optimal capacity. When anything is out of alignment, the body automatically goes to work to correct it. For example, the ideal temperature for a human body is 98.6° Fahrenheit. When we are 98.6° we are in homeostasis. When body temperature rises above this ideal, our body corrects the imbalance by releasing sweat, which cools us. As long as we have the water necessary in our system to produce this sweat, we are very effective at maintaining homeostasis.

If the connective tissue breaks down, our body innately knows that something is out of alignment—that we are no longer in homeostasis. It immediately goes to work to repair the irregular tissue, to rebuild it from its components. Our bodies are adept at rebuilding tissue as long as they have the parts available to them. Unfortunately, that is not always the case—which results in preventable disease, premature aging, and dimpling.

In Chapter 1 I mentioned that connective tissue was made up of the body's matrix, or substances called glycosaminoglycans or GAGs. To repair your connective tissue, you need to give your body the component part for this matrix—glucosamine. You also need to provide amino acids, the building blocks for collagen and elastin, which will keep your blood vessels firm and hold their shape. You need the vitamins and trace minerals necessary for your body to metabolize the amino acids and turn them into collagen and elastin. Finally, you need to give your body nutrients to rehydrate its blood vessels, to attract wasted water back to them—namely, essential fatty acids. Supplementing your diet with these nutrients may sound complicated at first, but it is actually very simple.

Vital Nutrients for Vibrant Skin

A patient I will call Emily came to see me about spider veins in her legs. Emily was in her late thirties when she first asked me to help her with this problem. She had grown up in Southern California, where she had a very active outdoor life and had been a professional beach volleyball player throughout her twenties. After she married and had her son, she stopped playing professionally, but she still regularly played with her friends. A few years ago, however, she began to notice spider veins on her thighs. She was embarrassed about showing her legs in public, and rather than playing volleyball in long pants, she stopped playing altogether. Finally she decided that something had to be done about it.

Every time Emily came to see me, I gave her a small injection of a saltwater solution that caused the vein to close up and eventually become absorbed into the body. It is a fairly effective method for dealing with the cosmetic problem of damaged blood vessels, and for a while it made her happy. She even began playing volleyball with her friends again. Whenever new veins appeared on her legs, she came to see me to have them cleared up. The problem with this treatment is that it doesn't target the cause of the condition, so it cannot prevent future spider veins from reappearing. Emily soon tired of new veins popping up, and the worst part was that they seemed to be reappearing with greater frequency. She felt that she couldn't see me fast enough to keep her legs clear of these blemishes. She once again stopped going to the beach. She became very upset at what was becoming a degenerative condition.

I wanted to prescribe a more long-term, all-encompassing solution for her. I asked myself how I could create an environment within Emily's body that would prevent the deterioration of blood vessels and the creation of spider veins. I asked myself,

What are blood vessels made of? The answer was obvious: connective tissue, collagen, and elastin—just like the skin's dermis.

The best solution was to put Emily on a diet that would give her blood vessels all of the nutrients they needed to get stronger on their own. I knew that if I could provide the building blocks for these three components of blood vessels, they would be able to regenerate and remain strong. It made sense that with the proper nutrition, her capillaries would stop dying and showing up as spider veins. This was an unconventional method of treatment, but I knew that if Emily gave it a chance, she would be thrilled with the results.

The body is like a tree. If it does not receive adequate water and sunlight, it will weaken. As soon as a parasite comes along, it will likely kill the tree no matter how much pesticide you put on it. However, if you give the tree all of the nutrients that it needs to stay healthy on its own, it may be strong enough to get rid of the disease by itself, without the help of pesticides. But even if not, the pesticides will be more likely to work to heal the disease state if the tree is healthy to begin with.

Before there was medicine, there was food.

Step 1. The Matrix

Unfortunately, it is not always easy for our bodies to obtain the necessary nutrients from food. As you know, connective tissue is made up of the body's matrix or GAGs. This includes chondroitin, dermatan and, most abundantly, hyaluronic acid. To make these substances, your body converts them from a nutrient called glucosamine. Your body does produce glucosamine, but not in sufficient amounts to replenish all of its connective tissue. In order for your body to be able to create new, healthy dermal tissue, it must be supplied with outside sources of this vital nutrient. Because glucosamine is not readily found in foods, I recommended that Emily start taking supplements, which are sold in any vitamin shop. A dosage of 1000 to 2000 mg a day is enough to supply your body's connective tissue with reinforcing GAGs.

Hyaluronic acid, one of the GAGs converted from glucosamine that make up the connective tissue, also attracts water to your tissues. It is found primarily in the joints, the eyes, and most plentifully in the skin. It is your body's natural moisturizer. This substance actually has the ability to hold one thousand times its weight in water. It is essential for keeping all of your connective tissue hydrated and therefore in a state of optimal health and vitality. As we age, our bodies produce less and less of this amazing substance, leaving us with sore joints and dry, wrinkly skin. Adding glucosamine, the building block of hyaluronic acid, to your diet will help your body's interior and exterior to stay moist and supple.

Step 2. Amino Acids

Emily also needed to supplement her diet with amino acids to build and repair the collagen and elastin in her blood vessels.

In general, our bodies can get the amino acids they need from our internal amino acid pool and from a diet that includes sufficient protein. When we eat protein-containing foods, our body breaks the protein down into various amino acids. It then absorbs these amino acids and rebuilds them into the sequence that we need for specific body tasks. Out of twenty amino acids, only eleven can be manufactured by our body. However, the body cannot function without all twenty amino acids, so it is essential that you get the remaining nine from food sources. Because of this, the nine amino acids our bodies cannot make are referred to as essential amino acids, and I wanted to make sure Emily was getting an adequate supply of these in order to fortify her muscles, connective tissue, and especially her collagen and elastin.

You may have heard that you can obtain all of the amino acids your body needs from meat. Yes and no. The amino acids in meat have already been converted into collagen and elastin in the animal's body. Your body needs to break down the animal's collagen and elastin into amino acids before it can make use of them. More direct sources of these nutrients are beans, whole grains, nuts, seeds, and vegetables and fruits, including my favorite superfood, goji berries. These plant foods are sources of protein that provide the body with adequate amounts of essential amino acids as long as a variety of them are consumed and your calorie needs are met. They contain amino acids that are much easier for your body to metabolize.

I recommended that Emily stick to a diet with a variety of quality protein sources such as plant foods and tofu, and replace red meat with omega-3 rich fish and skinless white meat poultry.

Step 3. Essential Fatty Acids

A successful diet to repair Emily's connective tissue also needed to include water attracters to reintroduce water into her blood vessels. The primary water attracters for connective tissue are essential fatty acids (EFAs), which are found in various seeds and nuts such as ground flaxseeds and walnuts, as well as in cold-water fish. Essential fatty acids are another superfood. They are loaded with health benefits, about which you will be hearing plenty more before this book is done. Unfortunately, your body is unable to produce these much-needed fats on its own, so you must get them from food sources or supplements. I asked Emily to take two 1000-mg fish oil EFA supplements every day. (A vegetarian alternative is four 1000-mg flaxseed oil EFA supplements plus 100–300 mg of a microalgae-derived DHA supplement.)

In addition to taking these EFA supplements, I told Emily to try to replace foods in her diet containing "bad" saturated and trans fats, such as red meat and margarine-containing hydrogenated fats, with foods containing "good" unsaturated fats, such as fish, canola oil, and olive oil. I did caution her to consume fats in moderation, however, as too much—even if it is good fat—can contribute to weight gain.

Step 4. B Vitamins and Trace Minerals

We also need specific nutrients to help us metabolize the glucosamine, amino acids, and EFAs into new, healthy connective tissue. These are the oil in the gears of the factory. They are B vitamins and trace minerals, including manganese, magnesium, copper, and zinc.

I recommend choosing a daily multivitamin/multimineral supplement that has at least 100 percent of the Daily Value (DV) for all eight of the B complex vitamins. This includes biotin, one of the most expensive vitamins, which some manufacturers skimp on providing.

DAILY B VITAMIN REQUIREMENTS

B Vitamin	100% DV
thiamine (B_1)	1.5 mg
riboflavin (B_2)	1.7 mg
niacin (B_3)	20 mg
pantothenic acid (B_5)	10 mg
pyridoxine (B_6)	2 mg

cobalamin (B$_{12}$)	6 mcg
folic acid	400 mcg
biotin	300 mcg

In addition to a multi-, you may also consider taking a high-potency B-50 B complex supplement. This typically has 50 mg of each B vitamin except for folic acid (this is kept at 400 mcg), B$_{12}$, and biotin.

I also recommend choosing a multivitamin/multimineral supplement that provides at least 100 percent of the DV of the important minerals and trace minerals. Daily Value is what our government says is a requirement, but we are finding that our bodies need more than the DV to address specific needs. Therefore, in many cases you should take more than the DV.

DAILY MINERAL REQUIREMENTS

Minerals	100% DV
magnesium	400 mg
iron*	18 mg
zinc	15 mg
copper	2 mg
manganese	2 mg
iodine	150 mcg

*Choose an iron-free multivitamin/multimineral supplement if you are post-menopausal.

Minerals	100% DV
chromium	120 mcg
molybdenum	75 mcg
selenium	70 mcg

It may be difficult to find a daily multivitamin/multimineral that has 100 percent of the DV for minerals such as magnesium or calcium because they would take a large amount of space in a tablet, making the tablet too large to swallow. For some of these minerals, higher levels may be optimal. There is no percentage DV established for other trace minerals such as silicon, boron, vanadium, nickel, and tin, so look for a multivitamin/multimineral that also includes these ultra–trace minerals.

I also discuss some foods containing these key nutrients in Chapter 5.

Rather than have Emily completely change her diet and begin consuming foods that are hard to find, I recommended that she take all of these vitamins, minerals, and nutrients in daily supplement tablets. In fact, these are the ingredients that I eventually put into Murad Youth Builder Supplements and now have in my Firm and Tone Dietary Supplement Pack, along with a daily supply of antioxidants and anti-inflammatories. Emily was skeptical at first. "Vitamins to cure spider veins?" she asked. I asked her to give it a try, and if she wasn't happy with the results in five weeks, we could always go back to the saline injections. "I'm miserable now," she said. "What do I have to lose?"

She called me only three weeks later, thrilled with the results. Her spider veins were significantly diminished. She called me again after five weeks, and they were almost all gone. But there was so much more. Her body felt firmer—not just on her thighs, but all over. The small bit of cellulite that she had on her backside, which she had given up on getting rid of years ago, was visibly reduced. Best of all, she was back on the volleyball court. She said that she had more energy while playing than she had in years.

Cellulite Stage 2: The Dermis

The first stage of cellulite, blood vessel deterioration, does not always lead to spider veins and visible damaged capillaries, so most women do not begin to treat it as early as Emily did, and it soon leads to dermal deterioration. As the dermis stops getting its supply of freshwater and nutrients from your blood vessels, it becomes dry and brittle, and begins to lose its resiliency. Weakened dermis is ripe for attacks from sunlight, cigarette smoke, and the countless other sources of damage we are exposed to every single day. The dermis, as well as the collagen and elastin bundles within it, breaks apart, allowing the dermal fat cells to push their way into this layer of connective tissue. By this point, cellulite is already visible when squeezed between your fingers, and you can feel its texture when you touch the affected areas.

Don't worry—there is a bright side. Your dermis is connective tissue just like your blood vessels. All of those nutrients that you need to take to repair your blood vessels are just as effective in repairing your dermis to prevent cellulite from becoming visible. My dermis-fortifying diet has even more benefits. Wrinkles also are the result of collagen and elastin deterioration. By taking supplements and eating foods rich in glucosamine, amino acids, essential fatty acids, B vitamins, and trace minerals, you fortify your collagen and elastin fibers, and reduce your wrinkles too.

PATIENT TESTIMONIAL

◆ ◆ ◆

Karen
Age: 29
Occupation: Customer service representative
Areas of concern: Hips and thighs

Personal testimony: I'm a working mom and don't have enough time to focus on myself, but I thought I'd try this because the cellulite really bugged me. I started using everything faithfully but then stopped using the body gel after a few days because I just didn't have time morning and night. I took the vitamins at breakfast and then again with dinner. That part was easy. I don't exercise, and I eat a lot of fast food with the kids, so it was a big surprise to hear my husband comment that my legs and thighs looked less dimply. He didn't even know that the vitamins were for that purpose! I noticed that my face even looked smoother. I didn't follow all of my instructions, and I even gained a couple of pounds over these two months, but I'm happy that my cellulite improved, and my husband noticed the change.

Clinical Program
- daily intake of supplements to address cellulite as outlined in this book
- topical application of cellulite serum

A few years ago, I wanted to examine this diet's effect on wrinkles, so I put together a study that would test the benefits of this program. I knew that the breakdown of connective tissue, collagen, and elastin that sets the stage for cellulite is the same deterioration that causes wrinkles. The primary function of those tissues in your skin is to keep it firm—both dimple- *and*

Clinical Results
Initial visit: stage-3 cellulite
Final visit: stage-2 cellulite

Additional Clinical Observations
Water measurements:
Visit 1 Intracellular 19.2 Extracellular 16.6
Visit 2 Intracellular 19.8 Extracellular 15.7
Final Intracellular 20.6 Extracellular 15.6
After 8 weeks there was a 1% decrease in extracellular water and a
1.4% increase in intracellular water.

% Body Fat
Visit 1: 42.2
Final visit: 35.2 (a decrease of 16.59%)

BMR (Basal Metabolic Rate, number of calories used at rest)
Visit 1: 1,351
Final visit: 1,481 (an increase of 130 calories burned per day at rest)

wrinkle-free. I knew that providing the body with all of the nutrients necessary for optimal dermal health would repair all of the effects of connective tissue breakdown. But I wanted proof.

We had the subjects in our study continue on their normal diets. Some of them added the supplements I prescribed, and some did not.

The experiment was a blinded study. That means that neither the subjects nor the researchers knew who was taking the nutrients. This eliminated the possibility of the researchers simply seeing what they wanted to see or what they thought they should see. We measured the subjects' wrinkles at the beginning of the study and after five weeks. The subjects taking the nutrients displayed a 34 percent reduction in their wrinkles in just five weeks!

Cellulite Stage 3: Your Visible Skin

Your epidermis, the upper portion of the skin, is your last line of defense against cellulite and stretch marks. When the cellulite has pushed through the dermis, it is visible only when it is squeezed. If the epidermis is damaged and weak, cellulite shows through it all of the time. As you now know, this layer of your skin is made of cells. If we are going to fortify this part of your body, we need to give it all of the nutrients that healthy cells need.

As I mentioned earlier, when cells sustain damage, their walls break apart and water seeps out. This causes them to become weak and inefficient. Superficially, this leads to dry, rough skin. These weakened cells can no longer hold fat invisibly beneath them. The fat that has broken through the dermal layer begins pushing closer to the skin cell layer of epidermis, where it becomes clearly visible cellulite. To prevent this, and to keep your skin smooth and supple, we need to replace the nutrients that the damaged cells have lost.

Lecithin and Lipids

The crumbling cell walls are made up of lecithin and lipids. Lecithin is found in many foods, predominantly egg yolks and soy. The best source of lipids to reinforce your cell walls are the same essential fatty acids that work so well reintroducing water to your dermis. As a bonus, these EFAs not only rebuild your cell walls, they also actually attract lost water back into your cells. A diet rich in lecithin and EFAs will do wonders hydrating your cells, thereby fortifying and strengthening the organs throughout your body. Cellulite is no match for cells fortified in such a way. Assuming they have not lost too much water, they will keep those unruly fat cells below your skin's surface where they belong. In addition to the essential fatty acids, I recommend adding lecithin-rich foods to your diet.

It is always preferable to get nutrients from foods. But if you do not regularly eat tofu, eggs, etc., it is important to take a supplement containing soy lecithin, or its building blocks, choline and phosphatidycholine, every day. Approximately 2000 to 4000 mg—or about the amount of found in a rounded tablespoon of soy lecithin granules or one large egg—is a good dosage to aim for.

Common Food Sources of Lecithin

soy foods (e.g., tofu)
soy lecithin granules
eggs
spinach
lettuce
cauliflower
peanuts and peanut butter
apples
oranges
potatoes

Unfortunately, most of us do not get the nutrients we need to keep our cell walls strong and have already lost plenty of our much-needed water. Aside from cellulite, we can feel the effects of this cellular water loss in many ways. For example, we are thirsty, even if we are drinking plenty of fluids. This is our cells sending us the message that they are dehydrated. We can try to feed them by drinking, but if their walls have lost integrity, the water will pass right through them—and right through us.

The water principle is a defining characteristic of health for your entire body. Dehydrated cells perform their duties far less efficiently than hydrated cells do. The cells that make up our liver, brain, heart, lungs, and every other organ cannot perform to their highest ability without the optimal amount of water. If your cells are in such a state you are likely to take far longer recovering from illness and infection than if you had hydrated cells. Dehydrated brain cells do not function at their optimal level, so you are likely to become mentally fatigued more easily. Your skin is likely dry and flaky. You have less energy and metabolize food less efficiently. Add to this the countless other deteriorating effects of cellular dehydration, including the advancement of cellulite, and you can begin to understand how critical it is to provide yourself with an ample supply of hydrating nutrients.

The Debilitating Effects of Water Loss

On weekends, I love to hike in the Santa Monica Mountains with my son and daughters. I've been hiking for years, and my stamina is pretty good. However, over time I began to notice that I ran out of steam earlier and earlier. I was getting fatigued at a fraction of the distances that I had once hiked with ease. I also noticed that I needed more water than I had in the past. On hikes I was parched. Drinking satisfied my thirst for only a brief period, and within minutes I needed to drink some more.

I knew that my body wasn't utilizing water as effectively as it once had, so I began making a conscious effort to eat more eggs, soy, fish, and nuts to rehydrate my body's tissues. In case I wasn't adding quite enough of these nutritional powerhouses to my diet, I took supplements of lecithin and EFAs every morning. Within weeks, I felt much more vibrant on my hikes. Soon afterward I noticed that I didn't need to carry a bottle of water with me, as my thirst no longer troubled me throughout the hike. I still had plenty of energy when I reached the end of trail, which summits at an overlook called Los Liones. It is a breathtaking view of a lush ravine, the beach, and the boundless Pacific Ocean flowing behind it. Sharing something so beautiful with my children is rejuvenating. It is the sort of experience that I live for.

With this hydrating diet, I had given vitality to my body's cells. My organs, my nervous system, my cardiovascular system, and everything else had been given an expert tune-up. If you begin to take the simple step of adding this short list of nutrients to your diet every day, not only will you see a drastic reduction in your cellulite and stretch marks, but your body will feel renewed too. It will function better, and it will be firmer to the touch. Because you can't always be sure if you are getting enough of each of them by just eating the right foods, I always tell my patients to take supplements as well. It does not harm you to take above the 100 percent DV of these substances. You can take these nutrients individually, or you can use the Murad Firm and Tone Dietary Supplement Pack that contains all of these ingredients in one pack.

Your skin, like the rest of your body, is designed to remain firm and youthful for years and years. All that it requires is regular maintenance. Think about it. When your body tells you that it wants food by creating hunger pains, you feed it, right? Signs such as cellulite, spider veins, and premature wrinkles are your body's way of telling you that your cells and connective tissue are hungry and thirsty. Go ahead, give them what they are craving. It couldn't be easier, and in a few weeks you will be thrilled with the results!

Dimple-Preventing Nutrients to Add to Your Diet
    antioxidants
    glucosamine
    amino acids
    essential fatty acids
    B vitamins
    trace minerals
    lecithin

◆

Four

Preventing Cellulite

You can prevent damage to your cells and connective tissue—which causes cellulite—from occurring in the first place. One of the most destructive effects of internal and environmental damage to our tissues is the creation of free radicals. These are rampaging cells in the body that start a chain reaction of damage. Damage strikes the body in many forms, including sunlight and pollution. In fact, a by-product of many of the body's own natural functions, such as breathing, is free-radical production. If we are to prevent the damage that leads to cellulite from happening, we must disarm free radicals.

Some Sources of Free-Radical Damage
UV radiation from the sun
pollution
cigarette smoke
stress/depression
lack of sleep

strenuous exercise

poor diet

Even day-to-day bodily functions such as breathing can produce free radicals

Free Radicals: The Agents of Aging

All of the molecules in our bodies are surrounded by pairs of
spinning electrons. In order for a molecule to be stable, it must
have an even number of these electrons. Even a single incomplete pair will cause that molecule to become thoroughly unbalanced. Free radicals are molecules in your body that have been
stripped of an electron by incoming damage.

As internal and external stresses strike our bodies, the first
thing they hit is the outer part of our cells—the cell walls. When
these forces attack a molecule in a cell wall, the result is the destruction of one of that molecule's electrons. One of its electron
pairs has now become incomplete, and it goes on a frantic search
for a partner. Its method is to crash about into all of its neighbors, damaging their electrons until it can finally steal one for itself and settle down again.

In the process of this destruction, each of the neighboring
molecules that has been crashed into and damaged by the original
one goes on its own rampage, causing the damage to spread like
wildfire. This spreading destruction is called oxidative stress. If
left unchecked, these growing masses of angry, incomplete molecules can lead to both visible and invisible aging, from wrinkles
to brain atrophy and even to cancer. The molecule that was first
attacked, the one that started this whole mess, is a free radical,
and each of the molecules that it damaged has itself become a
free radical, spreading its own teeming destruction. The only

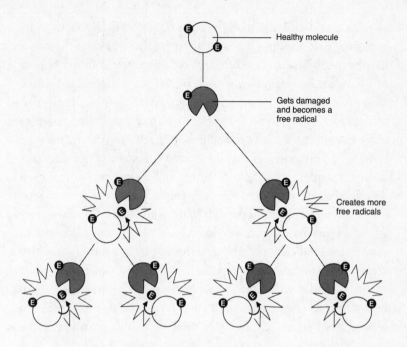

Healthy molecule

Gets damaged and becomes a free radical

Creates more free radicals

molecules that can lose electrons without becoming unstable are antioxidant molecules. They have the unique ability to stop oxidative stress in its tracks and thus are a vital component in a program to prevent the formation of cellulite.

Antioxidants: The Fountain of Youth

Antioxidants have been a hot topic in the health world for several years. You have likely heard much about the benefit and importance of antioxidants to your overall health. But you may not know what these age and disease fighters are and how they work.

Antioxidants are a wide range of naturally occurring substances that defend the body against damage. Each works in its own way and has its own special strengths. Individual antioxidants usually have an area of the body's tissues that they are most effective in. For example, ginkgo biloba seems to provide most of its benefit to the brain, while coenzyme Q_{10} is most effective in the heart. They come in a variety of forms, including vitamins and minerals. Some are created in your body, and others must be obtained from food and supplements. With state-of-the-art infusion techniques, some antioxidants, such as vitamin C, can even be effective when applied topically to the skin.

The one feature that they all share—the definitive characteristic that makes them antioxidants—is their unique ability to disarm free radicals, thereby preempting the spread of oxidative stress. Antioxidants are supplied with spare electrons. They travel around your system passing these out to free radicals in need. These graciously reformed free-radical molecules no longer need to assault and rob their neighbors in order to be complete.

The body naturally produces free radicals, and it also naturally produces antioxidants to disarm them. In this way it keeps oxidative stress in check. But because of the amount of free-radical damage inflicted on us from outside sources, our bodies do not produce sufficient quantities of antioxidants to counter it. The battle to keep cellulite at bay will ultimately be lost to the unchecked free radicals in our systems. In order to tilt the balance back in our favor, we need outside sources of antioxidants in the form of food and supplements. Cutting-edge scientific breakthroughs allowing certain antioxidants to penetrate into the deep layers of the skin have even allowed us to infuse free-radical fighters directly into our skin with creams applied topically. In this way we can have a reservoir of protection in our skin ready to be called upon at the first sign of damage.

Some Readily Available Antioxidant Sources

vitamin C: citrus fruits, goji berries

vitamin E: whole-grain breads, whole grains, nuts

vitamin A (beta-carotene): carrots and other orange and yellow fruits and vegetables

polyphenols: green tea, red and purple grapes, pomegranates

There are countless antioxidants available in food and in supplements. You don't need to take them all, but make sure you give your body an ample supply. There are many different kinds, each functioning best in a different part of the body. It is in your best interest to keep your body flooded with a variety of these antiaging miracles at all times. The best source is raw fruits and vegetables. In Chapter 5, you will read about my cellulite solution diet, which contains many more foods that are rich in healing, protective antioxidants. For now I'll go into detail on just a few of my favorites, the ones most effective at treating the free-radical damage that leads to cellulite.

Pomegranates: Symbols of Life

As I've said, before there was medicine, there was food. Pomegranate, one of the oldest medicines known, did much to improve the health of ancient people. It is mentioned in ancient Egyptian medical papyrus, and the ancient Greeks prescribed it as an anti-inflammatory and a cough suppressant, and for arteriosclerosis, asthma, and a host of intestinal disorders.

Pomegranates also occupy an important place in the art, literature, and folklore that shape our collective worldview. We can see them in the works of Cézanne and Dalí, in the Bible, and in Greek mythology. The pomegranate frequently symbolizes life and fertility. These ancient stories and medical texts were on to something. Pomegranates have amazing benefits to health and longevity. They are one of nature's most potent sources of polyphenols, a family of antioxidants that function primarily within the skin. Ellagic acid, which is found abundantly in pomegranates, is the most important polyphenol. It has the strongest age-proofing capabilities of any antioxidant examined to date, and studies at Northwestern University and the universities of Wisconsin and North Dakota have found pomegranate extract and ellagic acid to be powerful forces in the fight against cancer. According to a study published in the *Journal of Agriculture and Food Chemistry,* pomegranate juice has three times the antioxidant activity of green tea or red wine.

Since I began practicing medicine in 1972, I have been studying the ability of antioxidants to repair and protect the skin. The ellagic acid found in pomegranates is among the most recent additions to our arsenal of antioxidants. I was able to prove through an independent study that pomegranate extract boosts the SPF of sunscreen by 20 percent, and taking pomegranate internally before using sunscreen increases the SPF by 25 percent. This means that we can maintain the same level of protection against free radicals and inflammation from the sun using fewer chemicals and more antioxidants. Pomegranate is so effective at preventing sun damage that I added it to all of the products in my sun care line. In fact, I was so impressed with the results of the study that I created a supplement of pure pomegranate extract.

Due to its incredible antioxidant potency within the skin, ellagic acid is a vital ally in the fight against cellulite, which is unleashed by free-radical damage within the skin. For the ellagic acid benefit of this fruit, go right to the source. Pomegranates and pomegranate juice are a delicious way to protect your body. If these are in short supply in your local market, you can take a supplement containing pomegranate extract such as Murad Pomphenol Sunguard Supplement.

Vitamin C and Grape-Seed Extract

In addition to their remarkable antioxidant powers within the skin (and the rest of the body, for that matter), grape-seed extract and vitamin C break down substances in your body known as collagenase and elastase, which destroy the collagen and elastin in your connective tissue. This means that these antioxidants actually prevent the damage that directly causes sagging skin and wrinkles, and—you guessed it—opens the door to cellulite. These antioxidants fight a two-front battle against dimples—one against free radicals and one against connective tissue breakdown.

Goji Berries: Nature's Cellulite Assassins

Goji berries, found in Tibet and Inner Mongolia, might as well be called dimple-free berries. They are perhaps the most nutritionally dense food on the planet, the list of nourishing ingredients they contain reading like a who's who of cellulite elimination. Not only that, but their overall health benefits are truly remarkable. It is reported that in villages where goji berries are eaten daily, it is not uncommon for people to live to be well over one hundred.

For their antioxidant benefits, they have nearly five hundred times more vitamin C per ounce than oranges and more beta-carotene than carrots. They contain eighteen types of amino acids, twenty-one trace minerals, and vitamins B_1, B_2, and B_6. Goji berries are also rich in linoleic acid (an essential fatty acid) and beta-sitosterol (an anti-inflammatory). And they taste good. I recommend mixing them into shakes and smoothies, sprinkling them on salads, fat-free yogurt, soy yogurt, or whole-grain cereal, or just eating them on their own. You can find them for sale on many Web sites as well as in some markets in your nearest Chinatown.

Inflammation

Free-radical damage is a primary force in the tissue breakdown that leads to cellulite, but it is not the only one. It works in conjunction with another natural aging factor—inflammation.

Inflammation is a sign that your body is repairing damage. The damage that triggers inflammation is the same as that which causes free radicals. In fact, free-radical oxidation itself is a common trigger of inflammation. After an injury, infection, or sunburn, the affected area becomes red and swollen. It may also become warm to the touch. This is your body dilating its blood vessels to flood the affected areas with special anti-inflammatory nutrients.

The problem is that remaining in a state of such high alert for extended periods of time ultimately has a destructive effect on your body. Many of the substances your body releases in response to inflammation actually cause the free-radical damage and cell wall deterioration that they are attempting to prevent. For this reason, it is important to use soothing anti-inflammatory ingredients, both topically and internally, to calm inflammation before it can do more harm than good.

Fortunately, anti-inflammatories are widely available in a variety of foods and supplements. In fact, antioxidants can also be considered anti-inflammatories because they prevent the free-radical damage that leads to inflammation. Inflammation exists both internally and externally. While it is important to reduce inflammation using soothing topical treatments, it is equally important to take anti-inflammatories by mouth to prevent inflammation inside your body, particularly in the dermis.

Topical and Internal Anti-Inflammatories
>   arnica
>   aloe vera
>   allantoin
>   chamomile
>   zinc

The Stratum Corneum: Reinforcing Your Body Armor

The final method of protecting your body from the damage that leads to cellulite and opens the door to stretch marks is to rejuvenate and protect your primary defense against external forces. You recall that the stratum corneum is the outer layer of dead and dying cells in the epidermis. Even though it is only 0.015 millimeter thick, it is our main barrier against toxins attempting to get into our skin and water and nutrients attempting to get out. It is also our natural defense against damaging UV radiation from the sun. As you know, when we lose essential components in our skin, or allow the damage that causes free radicals and inflammation, our tissues weaken, giving ground to advancing cellulite. If we are to keep damage out and water in, we need our stratum corneum to be strong and vital.

The stratum corneum is like a brick wall. The dead and dying cells act as the bricks, and a lipid layer holding them in place functions as the mortar. As the cells in this layer get older (and therefore dryer), they lose their barrier function. Our bodies deal with this by constantly producing new skin cells that move toward the surface, forcing out the top, dying cells. In this way, the stratum corneum remains vital enough to competently protect us against damage and water loss.

Unfortunately, as we age, our rate of cell turnover decreases. The stratum corneum becomes packed with cells that just don't hold water. By the time we reach the age of twenty, and often before, it is necessary to give our skin some assistance.

Exfoliation: Uncovering a Younger You

The best way to reinforce this crucial barrier is through exfoliation: actively removing the dead, ineffectual cells on the surface, sending our body the signal to produce new ones. This ensures that our skin's surface is replete with young, hydrated, efficient cells.

The difference between a young cell and a dead cell is similar to the difference between a live leaf and a dead one. A live leaf has a smooth waxy finish that protects it from the elements. It is thick and strong. A dead leaf is thin and brittle. It has lost its waxy coating. A strong wind can rip it right off the tree and cause it to crumble. The same is true for dead skin cells. They have lost the integrity of their outer membrane. They are weak and dry, and can no longer function effectively. Young, hydrated cells make up a strong and supple barrier. For glowing, healthy skin, your stratum corneum needs to be filled with the youngest cells possible. Without exfoliation, old, dead cells build up, giving you a dull, sallow complexion and highlighting imperfections such as wrinkles on your face and cellulite on your body.

There are two primary methods of exfoliation: chemical and mechanical. Chemical exfoliation involves the topical application of agents such as alpha and beta hydroxy acids. These get between the skin cells in the stratum corneum and loosen the outermost cells, enabling them to fall off more readily. Mechanical exfoliation involves using a rough sponge such as a loofah, a dry skin brush with natural bristles, or a cleanser that contains gentle abrasive materials such as jojoba beads, salt, or ground apricot seed. Mechanical exfoliation every day or every other day before you bathe is an excellent way not only to stimulate blood flow and exfoliate your skin but also to increase your body's ability to absorb any topical cellulite remedy you put on after your bath or shower.

Alpha and Beta Hydroxy Acids

My favorite chemical exfoliators come from the family of hydroxy acids. These are sometimes known as fruit acids, as many of them are found naturally in fruits. For example, malic acid comes from apples, and glycolic acid is found in sugarcane. Cleopatra was famous for taking baths in sour milk. It may not sound very appealing, but the lactic acid in milk gave her skin a vibrant, youthful glow.

In the 1980s I was a pioneer in introducing hydroxy acids into topical skin care. They are now ubiquitous in all varieties of creams and cleansers, and are essential components in increasing the youthful radiance of millions of users around the world.

The two hydroxy acids that have the most benefit to skin exfoliation are glycolic acid and salicylic acid. For the face, these can reduce fine lines and wrinkles. I recommend using cleansers, treatment creams, and/or moisturizers containing one or both of these exfoliators. But use caution. Everyone's skin produces new cells at its own pace. It is important not to remove dead cells faster than your body can replace them. If you experience any irritation or redness while using these products, use a smaller amount, or decrease the frequency of use.

Remember, everyone's skin is different and reacts in its own way. Watch for the signals. Your skin will let you know if it needs more or less. It is also important to note that not all creams containing glycolic acid are equal. The purity of the acid and the vehicle that delivers it into your skin affect the efficacy of the product. I suggest that you use well-known brands, or find out if the company uses United States pharmaceutical grade (USP) ingredients. These may be slightly more expensive, but they are more effective and less likely to irritate than lesser-quality ingredients are. The law does not require that cosmetics contain ingredients of this grade, but the finest product lines insist on using them.

◆

Listen to your body. Listen to your skin.

Aside from their exfoliating abilities, another wonderful benefit of hydroxy acids is that they increase the penetration and effectiveness of other topical agents. When you use a moisturizer, another important defender of the stratum corneum, in conjunction with a hydroxy acid, it is able to penetrate deeper into the epidermis, increasing its hydrating and protective abilities.

Dry Skin Brushing

Dry skin brushing is one of the most effective exfoliating treatments for skin with cellulite and stretch marks. Not only does regular use of this technique remove old dead and dying cells around your body, it also increases the blood flow to the affected areas and stimulates the lymphatic system's ability to remove built-up toxins.

Dry skin brushing is a simple technique that can have amazing benefits if done regularly. You need a body brush with a long handle so that you can reach all affected areas. Also make sure that the brush has natural bristles, such as those made from goat, boar, or vegetables.

I recommend brushing your dry skin once a day, preferably before bathing. Sweep the brush once or twice over the problem areas toward the heart. For example, on the thighs and backside, brush upward. On the stomach, brush slightly more softly and in a circular clockwise direction. Complete your brushing session with a bath or shower followed by an application of a moisturizing, stimulating, nutrient-rich body cream such as the Murad Firm and Tone Serum.

Dry skin brushing is a triple-action method of treating your cellulite. First, it exfoliates, which stimulates the growth of young healthy skin cells and aids in the absorption of topical cellulite treatments that follow it. Second, it stimulates the blood vessels, and as we know, a lack of blood flow is the first symptom of cellulite accumulation. And finally, skin brushing stimulates the lymphatic system. It is the job of the lymph nodes to aid in the removal of wastes and toxic substances throughout the body. As we age, the lymphatic system slows down and needs a bit of help to successfully complete its job. Dry skin brushing is an excellent way to achieve this. If you brush before a shower, don't use any mechanical or chemical exfoliants in the shower, as too much exfoliation can irritate the skin.

Moisturizers: Agents That Attract Water and Prevent Water Loss

You know how important it is to keep adequate moisture in your skin. One of the primary functions of the stratum corneum is to prevent the water within your skin from escaping. It is analogous to the roof of your house. When it is cold outside we put the heat on. But what happens if there are holes in the roof? The heat seeps right through it, leaving you cold even though you are inside.

The stratum corneum functions in much the same way. You

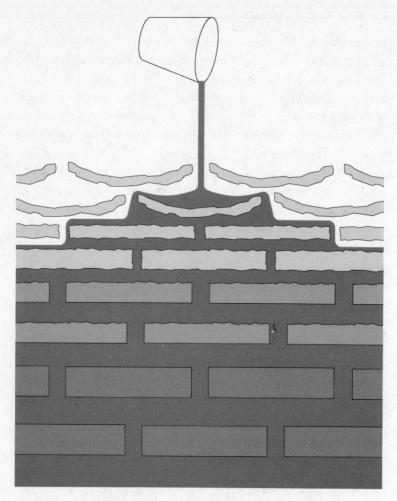

Stratum corneum improved by adding hydrating agents

can think of it as the roof of your body's house and your skin's vital water as the heat that is in danger of escaping. When we are young, this roof is firm and intact. As long as we are taking the right nutrients to put water in our skin, our stratum corneum provides a sturdy barrier to keep it there. Unfortunately, as we age, its barrier ability diminishes. Not only does it become filled with more dead, ineffectual cells than young, strong ones, the lipid layer that forms the seal between the cells becomes depleted. This leaves us ripe for what is called transepidermal water loss. Water escapes from our skin tissue and flows right through the stratum corneum and into the environment, much like heat escaping through holes in a weathered roof. Many people have dehydrated skin to begin with, ripe for opportunistic cellulite and stretch marks. And the limited water supply in their skin may be escaping right under their noses.

This explains why using a moisturizer is so important. Not only does a good moisturizing cream infuse skin with water, it reinforces the seal between the cells in your stratum corneum, preventing your vital water from running off and taking your skin's ability to fend off cellulite away with it.

The sealant ability of the stratum corneum is the result of two different kinds of substances. The first group is hydrophobic agents, elements that repel water. That may sound confusing. Why are we repelling water? Don't we want to attract water to our skin? Yes, we do, but we also want to prevent it from escaping in the first place. These elements repel the water that is trying to sneak out and push it back inside your tissues. Examples of hydrophobic elements in your skin are a class of lipids known as ceramides.

The other group of substances that give the stratum corneum its barrier ability is hydrophilic agents. These are water-loving materials that attract water from the environment and draw it into the skin. Examples of hydrophilic agents are sodium PCA and hyaluronic acid. A good moisturizer contains both kinds of hydrating substances to mimic and strengthen the stratum corneum. When applied to dry and damaged surface skin, they can reinforce the barrier function by filling in and reinforcing the tattered tissue. In this way they bolster the skin's protective coating, preventing transepidermal water loss and denying entrance to unwanted attackers.

Moisturizers perform another important function. While the deeper layers of our skin need to be hydrated from the inside by drinking water and ingesting hydrating nutrients, our stratum corneum has the unique ability to absorb hydration applied directly to it. Applying a moisturizer containing ingredients such as sodium PCA and hyaluronic acid can instantly and directly rehydrate and refortify your surface skin, making it a more potent force in preventing cellulite. It will look more beautiful and feel smoother too. The hydrating effects of topical moisturizers are temporary, but frequent and consistent application will maintain a healthy, hydrated environment in which the skin can flourish.

An Apple a Day

I point out to my patients that while our roofs help to keep heat in our houses, they have another important function as well. They protect us from the elements. Just as a damaged roof allows rain to leak in, a damaged stratum corneum allows the entrance of parasites and infection looking to attack your skin tissues.

A good analogy is to imagine that your body is an apple and the stratum corneum is the skin around it. If you cut an apple in half and leave it out and exposed to the elements, it turns brown and wrinkles. This is free-radical damage. Without skin to protect it from the environment, sunlight and toxins can directly attack its tissues. The same thing happens if you simply bruise an apple. Even though the skin looks like it is still intact, tiny holes in it have damaged its integrity where it was bumped. The area directly under the bruised skin also begins to turn brown and dry out.

In much the same way, the body's tissues, without proper protection and antioxidants, also become damaged, discolored, dehydrated, and wrinkled. If you squeeze a small amount of lemon juice on an apple that has turned brown, it turns a healthy white again. The high concentration of the antioxidant vitamin C in the lemon juice counteracts the free-radical damage done to the apple.

Another thing you notice is that even an intact apple shrinks and shrivels up after it has been sitting out for some time. This is because the free-radical damage to it has allowed the apple's vital water to escape in much the same way that water escapes from your body's tissues if they are not properly taken care of. In fact, even if we don't bruise or cut the apple, eventually the environment will take its toll and slowly break through the skin. If we put a protective coating of petroleum jelly around the apple, it would significantly delay the time it takes for the apple to go bad—especially if we included hydrating agents, antioxidants, and anti-inflammatories to this coating. A moisturizer applied to your skin functions in the same way and has the same clearly visible preventative antiaging properties.

I recommend applying a moisturizing cream every day to any area of your body that needs it, especially to areas where there is cellulite or where cellulite is likely to occur, such as your thighs and backside. An ideal moisturizer contains hydrators, antioxidants, and anti-inflammatory agents. (Indeed, I believe that all skin health products should include a combination of these healing agents.) This trifecta is the Murad recipe that is the foundation for all of my products. A moisturizer that is used to treat cellulite ideally also includes an agent that increases blood flow, such as cayenne or capsaicin.

It is also important to avoid actively drying out your surface skin by using harsh products or overcleansing. Use gentle products as much as possible. If your skin is feeling dry or irritated, switch to a moisturizing soap. Rubbing your skin dry with a towel strips your skin of necessary water and natural lipids. When you get out of the bath or shower, pat yourself dry and then immediately apply a moisturizer to trap the remaining water into your skin.

INGREDIENTS TO LOOK FOR IN A MOISTURIZER

Hydrators	Antioxidants	Anti-inflammatories
sodium PCA	vitamin C	zinc
hyaluronic acid	vitamin E	licorice extract
glycerine	pomegranate extract	aloe vera
goji berry extract	goji berry extract	goji berry extract

Sun Protection

By now it should come as no surprise to anyone how damaging to our skin the ultraviolet rays from the sun are. Not only does direct sunlight lead to dry skin, wrinkles, and hyperpigmentation, it is also one of the leading causes of free-radical damage that weakens skin cells and connective tissue. It is of primary importance in avoiding this cellulite-causing damage that you apply a broad-spectrum sunscreen to any part of your body that is exposed to direct sunlight. "Broad-spectrum" means that it protects you from the shorter "burning" UVB rays, and also the longer, more deeply penetrating "aging" UVA waves.

The best defense against cellulite is the prevention of the forces that cause it. The more we can minimize the free-radical production, inflammation, and resulting water loss, the less chance that new cellulite will ever form on our bodies. Combine this with the wonderful way you will be looking and feeling with all of these preventative nutrients, and I guarantee you will be thrilled with the results.

Extra Ingredients to Look for in Topical Products

    pomegranate extract (punica granatum extract)
    vitamin C
    grape-seed extract
    goji berries (lycium barbarum fruit extract)
    zinc
    carnitine
    arnica
    cat's-claw (uncaria tomentosa extract)
    cayenne (capsicum frutescens fruit extract)
    centella asiatica extract
    tiger's herb (centella asiatica extract)

PATIENT TESTIMONIAL

◆ ◆ ◆

Lucia
Age: 40
Occupation: Sales
Areas of concern: Outer thighs

Personal testimony: I had a few areas that I call dents in my outer thighs. Basically, they looked like deep grooves. This was really annoying, and when I pinched the area it looked really bad. I had lots of purple spider veins in the area also and had had them for years. I did ten endermology treatments and tried other creams, but they seemed to stop working when I stopped doing it. I stopped taking my daily vitamin and switched to these vitamins. After two weeks, I noticed the deep dents filling in, and the small purple veins started to disappear. Then I went on vacation and stopped taking the pills altogether. What a difference it made in my progress! I'm now taking them regularly and am applying the gel every day. My forty-five-year-old husband is in great shape but wanted a smoother abdomen. I've got him using the pills and the gel, and we are both noticing an improvement; he says his skin is less bloated. While I did not change my diet completely, I modified it to include more raw vegetables and replaced butter with olive oil. It's been easy. Both my husband and I are hooked.

Clinical Program
- daily intake of supplements to address cellulite as outlined in this book
- topical application of cellulite serum
- eat more fresh raw vegetables; switch from butter to olive oil

Clinical Results
Initial visit: stage-2 cellulite
Final visit: stage-1 cellulite

Additional Clinical Observations
Water measurements:
Visit 1 Intracellular <u>19.2</u> Extracellular <u>16.4</u>
Visit 2 Intracellular <u>18.3</u> Extracellular <u>16.0</u>
Final Intracellular <u>19.8</u> Extracellular <u>16.0</u>

% Body Fat
Visit 1: 34.7
Final visit: 32.9 (a decrease of 5.19%

BMR (Basal Metabolic Rate, number of calories per day used at rest)
Visit 1: 1,407
Final visit: 1,451 (an increase of 44 calories burned at rest)

◆

Five

The Youth-Building Cellulite Solution Diet

Don't let the name of this chapter scare you. The diet in my program is not about losing weight or depriving yourself of foods you love. It is about adding healthy foods that are rich in the seven cellulite-fighting nutrients to your diet. This is a modification of the Murad Method diet for health and vitality and is based on the water principle. What I ask you to do in this diet is introduce a wide variety of healthy, delicious foods into your regular routine and, whenever possible, substitute these for less healthy options. There is no need to strictly monitor your eating habits or make difficult sacrifices. All that I ask is that you incorporate these cellulite busters into your normal diet as much as you can. Because it is not always possible to eat enough of these foods, it is important also to take these nutrients in the form of supplements every day.

While shedding pounds is not the goal of this diet, if you are overweight, weight loss is certainly in your best interest. Adding the specific foods that I recommend will target and repair your cellulite and stretch marks, but they will not work as well if you are not as healthy as you can be. Health breeds health. Any program will have to work harder and will be less successful when it is up against an out-of-shape, overweight body. The following foods, when eaten in moderation, will give your body the tools that it needs to become and remain healthy without contributing to weight gain. People who have gone on this diet boast of having more energy, getting sick less frequently, and having firmer skin. They also came away with a lower body fat percentage and a higher basal metabolic rate. That means that their bodies burned more calories than before the program without adding any extra activity to their routine. You probably thought you'd never hear anyone say this, but you can smooth out your cellulite by eating!

Cellulite Stopper #1: Lecithin

Lecithin is a vital component to any cellulite elimination program. Lecithin repairs tissues by filling in and rebuilding cell walls, helping all of your organs to be fully hydrated and function at their highest level. The visible effect of this is lustrous, youthful skin that is too strong for cellulite to show through it.

Food Sources of Lecithin

> eggs
>
> soy products, including tofu, soy milk, and soy cheese. (These may be a better choice than eggs, as they have no cholesterol. If you have concerns about the cholesterol found in eggs, you can consider taking soy lecithin supplements such as cholesterol-free powdered soy lecithin granules,

which can be added to your favorite foods and beverages. one tablespoon of soy lecithin granules has 1725 mg of lecithin.)

cauliflower

peanuts and peanut butter

oranges

potatoes

spinach

iceberg lettuce

tomatoes

In order to ensure that you are getting enough of this cell-hydrating powerhouse, take a lecithin supplement (2000–4000 mg) every day.

Cellulite Stopper #2: Glucosamine

As your body sustains damage, your skin's dermis breaks down. A damaged dermis cannot maintain sufficient water content and begins to dry out and break apart. This leaves your skin with a loss of elasticity, wrinkles, and cellulite. Weak, brittle connective tissue is easily overrun with dermal fat cells, causing dimples in the skin. Unfortunately, your body does not produce enough of the component parts to make new connective tissue to repair dermis as quickly as it is damaged. Glucosamine is the building block for the ingredients needed to repair the dermis—as well as all of the rest of the connective tissue throughout your body. An adequate supply of this rejuvenating skin strengthener may be the most important component of a cellulite-fighting plan.

Glucosamine is not readily found in foods (unless you want to start eating unpeeled shrimp). It is available as a supplement on its own or as part of a multinutrient in any vitamin store. Take 1200 mg of either glucosamine sulfate or glucosamine hydrochloride (HCL) every day.

Cellulite Stopper #3: Essential Fatty Acids

Every part of the body—the brain, the heart, the lungs, the skin, the muscles and ligaments, and everything else for that matter—needs water to function properly. Without enough water in their cells, organs cannot perform their normal operations or communicate with each other. As you know, water loss within the cells and connective tissue is associated with health problems in all of the body's systems. Yet as we age, our cells and connective tissues hold on to less and less water. Or is it that as we lose the ability to hold onto water, we age?

There is a family of substances that not only attracts water to dehydrated cells and connective tissue all throughout our bodies but also prevents future water loss by repairing our cell walls. Essential fatty acids are the oil that lubricates the body's gears. I can't say enough good things about them. In fact, the only thing wrong with them is that they are not naturally produced within the human body. To obtain essential nutrients that make up the essential fatty acids, we need to go to outside sources.

Omega-3 fatty acids contain alpha linoleic acid; omega-6 fatty acids contain linoleic acid and gamma linoleic acid. Take at least 2.2–4.4 g of alpha linoleic acid (omega-3 fatty acid) per day. Although omega-6 fatty acid is also important, it is much more prevalent in the average American diet, so we generally don't need to take those supplements. Also replace foods that contain unhealthy saturated and trans fats in your diet with foods that contain EFAs, as well as other healthy unsaturated fats such as oleic acid (omega-9 fatty acid). Olive oil is rich in oleic acid. Cold-water fish are the best animal source of omega-3 fatty acids and flaxseeds are one of the best plant sources.

Unhealthy Fats
butter
margarine
partially hydrogenated vegetable oils or vegetable shortening
potato and other deep-fried chips
fat in beef and pork

EFAs and Other Healthy Fats
flaxseed oil
olive oil
canola oil
walnut oil
seeds (ground flaxseeds, sunflower seeds, hemp seeds)
nuts (raw walnuts, almonds, cashews, Brazil nuts, pistachios)
oil from cold-water fish

Some of these fish, such as tuna and salmon, can contain high levels of mercury and other contaminants, so you should eat these infrequently. Women who are pregnant or breast-feeding should limit tuna to once every two to three weeks. EFA supplements are the safest and surest way to get your daily allowance of this wonder nutrient.

As a general rule, some fish are safe to eat every day, while others are more of a concern. When deciding what to have for dinner, use this guide as a reference.

Best Choice	Caution	Avoid
abalone (farmed)		
anchovy		
bigeye (troll or poll caught)		
catfish (U.S., farmed)		
caviar (farmed)		caviar (beluga, osetra, sevruga)
clams (farmed)	clams (wild caught)	
cod (black/Alaska, British Columbia)	cod (Pacific, black/ Washington, Oregon, California)	cod (Atlantic, Icelandic, rock)
crab (Dungeness)	crab (snow, imitation/surimi, king/Alaska)	crab (king/imported)
halibut (Pacific)		
herring		
hoki		
		lingcod
lobster (rock/ California, Australia)	lobster (American)	
mackerel		
	mahimahi	

Best Choice	Caution	Avoid
		monkfish
mussels (farmed)	mussels (wild caught)	
		orange roughy
oysters (farmed)	oysters (wild caught)	
	pollack	
		rockfish
sablefish (Alaska, British Columbia)	sablefish (Washington, Oregon, California)	
salmon (canned, wild caught Alaska, California)	salmon (wild caught Washington, Oregon)	salmon (Atlantic farmed)
	sand dabs	
sardines		
	scallops (bay farmed, sea)	
sea bass (white)		sea bass (Chilean)
	shark (thresher U.S. West Coast; the Audubon Society lists all shark in its "many problems" category)	shark (all other)

Best Choice	Caution	Avoid
shad		
shrimp/prawns (trap caught; the Audubon Society lists all shrimp in its "many problems" category)	shrimp (U.S. farmed or wild)	shrimp (imported)
		snapper (Pacific)
	sole (English, petrel, Dover, rex)	
squid (California)		
sturgeon (farmed)		sturgeon (wild caught)
	swordfish (U.S. West Coast)	swordfish (Atlantic)
tilapia (farmed)		
	trout (rainbow farmed)	
tuna (albacore, yellowfin)	tuna (albacore, yellowfin, bigeye longline or purse-seine caught; canned)	tuna (bluefin)

Sources: Monterey Bay Aquarium Seafood Watch and the Audubon Society Seafood Lover's Guide.

Cellulite Stopper #4: Amino Acids

You are probably more familiar with the term "protein" than "amino acids." Protein is made up of the twenty amino acids that we need to rebuild damaged tissue and for our body's day-to-day functions. When we eat protein-rich foods, our bodies break them down into individual amino acids. Among the myriad reasons amino acids are important is that they are essential in the production of collagen and elastin within the body's connective tissue.

While all of these amino acids are essential, only nine of them are actually called "essential amino acids." Even though we need all twenty to function, our body cannot manufacture these nine on its own. We need to obtain them from outside food sources.

Essential Amino Acids
    histidine
    isoleucine
    leucine
    lysine
    methionine
    phenylalanine
    threonine
    tryptophan
    valine

Nonessential Amino Acids
    alanine
    arginine
    asparagine
    aspartic acid
    cysteine

glutamic acid
glutamine
glycine
proline
serine
tyrosine

All meat, poultry, fish, cheese, milk, eggs, and soy contain good amounts of all nine essential amino acids. Leafy green vegetables, nuts, and wheat also contain protein. A well-balanced diet with a variety of protein sources is likely to give you all the nine essential amino acids that you need. (Vegetarians may also want to add a spoonful of soy protein isolate powder to their diet every day. You can mix this into cereal or fat-free yogurt, or even bake with it.) The average recommended daily protein allowance for women is approximately 50 g per day.

Cellulite Stopper #5: Antioxidants

Without antioxidants we would succumb to disease and aging years before our time. Giving your body an ample supply of healing antioxidants is the only way to stop free-radical damage from ravaging all of its tissues. They are so effective at preventing damage that many are even widely used to help prevent cancer. Among their many functions in the skin is their ability to prevent the damage that weakens your dermis and epidermis and opens the door to cellulite. Enough antioxidants in your diet can prevent tissues from breaking down and turning into future lumps and dimples.

While some antioxidants have a recommended daily allowance, such as vitamins A, C, and E, most do not. When you are on this diet, don't try to count milligrams of your antioxidant intake. Basically, get as many of these age-preventing all-stars in your diet as possible.

The best sources of antioxidants are plants. While berries and citrus fruits are the most plentiful sources, all fruits and vegetables provide good supplies of antioxidants. As a general rule, the darker and brighter the color of the food, the more densely packed with vitamins it is. Blueberries are a great example. The rich blue coloring of this fruit is a hint of its strong concentration of free-radical-fighting flavonoids. The next time you are in the produce aisle, see what immediately grabs your eye. It is likely the most beneficial. Buy the most vivid, luscious-looking fruit you can find. Your body will thank you.

Another helpful antioxidant hint is to avoid cooking these foods too much. The more heat they are subjected to, the more vital nutrients and water are lost. In most cases, raw fruits and vegetables have the strongest concentration of antioxidants. Also, eat foods that are as fresh as possible. The longer these foods are off the tree or vine, the more the antioxidants within them dissipate.

Polyphenols

Polyphenols are my favorite family of antioxidants. These are a class of plant chemicals found in high concentrations in tea, red grapes, red wine, and many other foods that are associated with cancer prevention, reducing heart disease, and skin health. The strongest polyphenol is ellagic acid. The highest levels are found in raspberries, strawberries and, of course, pomegranates.

Polyphenol Food Sources
    nuts
    whole-grain cereals
    brightly colored fruits, vegetables, berries
    soybeans

> tea (especially green tea)
> red grapes
> red wine
> onions
> citrus fruits
> pomegranates
> goji berries

Vitamin A

Vitamin A is an antioxidant that plays a large role in the repair of body tissues and is vital for good eyesight and healthy skin.

Vitamin A Food Sources
> liver
> sweet potatoes
> carrots
> goji berries
> mangoes
> eggs
> milk

Vitamin C

Citrus fruits and goji berries are the best source of vitamin C. However, virtually all fruits and vegetables contain this potent antioxidant.

Other Sources of Vitamin C
> kiwi
> mango
> papaya
> black currants

Vitamin E

Vitamin E is a very potent fat-soluble antioxidant. This means that it can be stored in your cell walls, ready for immediate protection from free radicals. Vegetable oils, nuts such as almonds, wheat germ, and dark green leafy vegetables are the best food sources of vitamin E. The RDA of vitamin E is 15 mg or 22 IU.

Other Healing Antioxidants

There are countless antioxidants available. In addition to eating antioxidant-rich foods as often as possible, take an antioxidant supplement every day that contains some or all of these nutrients.

Antioxidants to Look for in Supplements
   vitamins A, C, E
   citrus bioflavonoids
   green tea extract
   grape-seed extract
   pomegranate extract
   goji berry extract
   poria cocos
   milk thistle
   n-acetyl cysteine
   rosemary leaf extract
   yellow dock root
   quercetin
   curcumin (turmeric)
   ginkgo biloba
   selenium
   coenzyme Q_{10}

Cellulite Stopper #6:
Anti-inflammatories

The next step in reducing your cellulite is simple. An anti-inflammatory diet is one that is stocked with antioxidant-rich, brightly colored fruits and vegetables, and plenty of healthy protein-incorporating omega-3 and omega-9 fatty acids. Who would have guessed that soothing your tissues and smoothing your thighs could be so delicious?

While a general anti-inflammatory diet is the ideal way to prevent the damage that results from inflammation, there are a few specific food ingredients that are ceaseless inflammation stoppers.

Alpha Linoleic Acid

Alpha linoleic acid (ALA) is found in many common foods, including vegetables, beans, fruits, in a concentrated form in flaxseed oil, as well as in canola, wheat germ, and walnut oils (including raw walnuts). It is in the omega-3 family of fatty acids, so fish oils also are included as an ALA anti-inflammatory oil.

Sources of ALA
> lettuce
> broccoli
> spinach
> navy, pinto, and lima beans,
> peas and split peas

Gamma Linoleic Acid

Gamma linoleic acid (GLA) is the other super inflammation-soothing food. It is a more rare oil, found in seed oils such as borage oil, evening primrose oil, black currant oil, and hemp oil.

Whenever possible, substitute pro-inflammatory foods with these soothing anti-inflammatories.

Inflammatory Foods	Anti-inflammatory Alternatives
red meat	cold-water fish
butter	olive oil
cheese	tofu, soy cheese
snacks loaded with saturated or trans fats	seeds, nuts, fresh and natural dried fruits (including goji berries)
foods loaded with simple sugars, such as cookies, candies, cakes	fresh fruits and vegetables

Food for Thought

Every cell in your body needs sodium to work properly. It is essential for the healthy function of nerve and muscle, including your heart muscle. The problem with sodium is that most of us consume far more than we need. Since your body requires a certain balance of sodium and water at all times, extra salt requires extra water, which results in water retention. Instead of using salt and pepper, try seasoning your meals with anti-inflammatory herbs such as basil, oregano, rosemary, garlic, and ginger.

In addition to these easy dietary changes, I recommend taking a daily supplement containing these other anti-inflammatory ingredients:

- arnica
- chamomile
- EFAs
- licorice extract
- vitamin E
- zinc

Cellulite Stopper #7:
B Vitamins and Trace Minerals

All of the nutrients I've mentioned so far are invaluable tools in keeping cellulite at bay. However, they do you no good at all if your body is not able to metabolize them into smooth skin and firm connective tissue. The nutrients necessary for this task are the B complex vitamins and trace minerals.

B Vitamins

There are eight B vitamins. The majority of our B vitamin needs can be met with healthy food sources such as brewer's (nutritional) yeast, wheat germ, whole grains, beans, dark green vegetables, low-fat and nonfat dairy products, fish, eggs, and poultry.

FOOD SOURCES FOR B VITAMINS

vitamin B_1 (thiamine)	brewer's yeast, sunflower seeds, wheat germ, green peas, whole grains, beans
vitamin B_2 (riboflavin)	low-fat and nonfat dairy products, dark green leafy vegetables, brewer's yeast, asparagus, broccoli, whole grains

niacin	poultry, fish, mushrooms, nuts, brewer's yeast, green peas, whole grains, beans
vitamin B$_6$ (pyridoxine)	watermelon, bananas, spinach, soybeans, brewer's yeast, fish, poultry, wheat germ, whole grains
folate (folic acid)	brewer's yeast, dark green leafy vegetables, asparagus, orange juice, beets, broccoli, beans
vitamin B$_{12}$	fish, poultry, low-fat and nonfat dairy products, fortified soy milk, eggs, nutritional yeast
biotin	eggs, most vegetables, brewer's yeast, wheat germ, oatmeal, cereals, almonds, soybeans, bananas, grapefruit, tomatoes
pantothenic acid	all plant and animal foods; especially salmon, chicken, avocado, mushrooms, sweet potatoes, low-fat and nonfat milk, eggs, soybeans, peanut butter, bananas, oranges, whole grains

While we do get most of these in our daily food intake, it is advisable to take a supplement with a B complex daily to ensure optimal metabolism.

PATIENT TESTIMONIAL

◆ ◆ ◆

Laura
Age: 44
Occupation: Office manager
Areas of concern: Thighs and buttocks

Personal testimony: At age forty-four, I knew my body needed some extra attention. Even though I exercised, ate right, and was in pretty good shape, I wanted to try something for the stubborn cellulite on the back of my thighs and bottom. Since I live near the beach, I wanted to feel good in a swimsuit again. I'm also in a new relationship, which makes me more self-conscious about these areas. I did leg lifts every day and rode my bike to get rid of it, and it did not budge. So when I started this program I promised myself to try everything they recommended. I applied the gel, took the vitamins, ate the foods they suggested, and did a series of firm-and-tone spa treatments. After only two months I have seen a great improvement. I wore a bikini, and I have to say I love the results! It was totally worth it and I will continue to stay on it forever. Thank you!

Clinical Program
- daily intake of supplements to address cellulite as outlined in this book

Trace Minerals

Trace minerals are so called because we need only trace amounts of them to feel their benefits. Because so little is needed, it is easy to receive an ideal daily allowance of these nutrients from

- topical application of cellulite serum
- reduce red meat, eat more soy, drink pomegranate juice, eat goji berries
- dry brushing of skin
- professional spa body-firming treatments

Clinical Results
Initial visit: stage-3 cellulite
Final visit: stage-1 cellulite

Additional Clinical Observations
Water measurements:
Visit 1 Intracellular 15.4 Extracellular 12.8
Visit 2 Intracellular 16.3 Extracellular 13.4
Final   Intracellular 16.1 Extracellular 12.1

% Body Fat
Visit 1: 26.0%
Final visit: 20.3 (a decrease of 21.9%)

BMR (Basal Metabolic Rate, number of calories used per day at rest)
Visit 1: 1,223
Final visit: 1,303 (an increase of 80 calories burned at rest)

our diets. However, as a deficiency of trace minerals can result in all manner of problems, including heart disease, a weakened skeletal system, and protein deficiencies, it is important to take trace mineral supplements daily.

Trace Minerals
zinc
copper
selenium
magnesium
boron
chromium
manganese
molybdenum
silica
vanadium

Healthy Eating for a Healthy Body

In addition to eating foods containing the specific nutrients that directly eliminate cellulite, it is necessary to create an environment of inclusive health within your body. Your system will find it easier to smooth out the imperfections in your skin if it is also running smoothly internally.

Having a healthy mental state is another vital step in repairing any affliction in your body. That is why I have made the cellulite diet easy. An unnecessarily strict diet that causes undue stress eventually winds up doing more harm than good, and it is unlikely that you will stick to it.

Five Tips for Healthy Eating
1. Eat when you are hungry, not when you think you should eat.
2. Stop eating when you are full, not when your plate is empty.

3. Listen to your body. We often get cravings for foods rich in nutrients that we are deficient in.
4. Substitute healthy alternatives and cellulite-stopping foods whenever possible.
5. Take supplements every day.

Smoothies are an excellent energy booster and a great breakfast option or midafternoon snack. For best flavor and smooth consistency, drink them as soon as you have made them. Experiment with different fruits, juices, and spices. Dried fruits offer another good option when your favorite fresh fruits are not in your local market.

The Murad Seven-Day Cellulite Solution Sample Meal Plan

Below is a sample week-long meal plan. Try incorporating a few of these ideas at a time. There is no need to strictly follow this plan. Just use it to give yourself some ideas. However, the more you follow these dietary guidelines, the more successful you will be.

Day 1

Breakfast

Murad Cellulite Solution Smoothie*
½ large grapefruit
2 slices whole-grain toast with sugar-free fruit jam
decaffeinated coffee or caffeine-free herbal or green tea

*Recipe is provided. See page 110.

Midmorning Snack

1 cup red, purple, or black grapes
1 hard-boiled egg or 1 cup soy milk

Lunch

tossed green salad with Fat-Free Oriental or Vinaigrette
    dressing* or Flax-Goji Golden Citrus Dressing*
1 cup Chicken-Vegetable Soup* or Vegetarian Split Pea with
    Barley Soup*
2–4 Scandinavian-type whole-grain rye crackers
iced caffeine-free herbal or green tea or mineral water with
    lime

Midafternoon Snack

1 cup raw vegetables with optional fat-free dressing for dip
6 raw almonds

Dinner

vegetable salad with extra-virgin Olive Oil and Lemon Juice
    Dressing*
Steamed Vegetables with Low-Fat Marinara Sauce*
medium baked potato with 1 teaspoon flaxseed oil and herb
    seasoning
mineral water with lime or caffeine-free herbal or green tea

Dessert

½ cup fat-free, sugar-free plain yogurt or soy yogurt topped
    with ½ cup fresh or unsweetened frozen strawberry
    slices

*Recipe is provided. See pages 110–114.

Day 2

Breakfast

Murad Cellulite Solution Smoothie
½ cup old-fashioned oatmeal with cinnamon and fat-free milk or soy milk
⅓ medium or 1 cup cubed cantaloupe
decaffeinated coffee or caffeine-free herbal or green tea

Midmorning Snack

1 medium orange
4 raw walnuts

Lunch

vegetable salad with fat-free dressing
1 cup lentil soup
whole wheat roll
apple
iced caffeine-free herbal or green tea or mineral water with lemon

Midafternoon Snack

1 cup raw vegetables with optional fat-free dressing for dip
1 cup fat-free milk or soy milk or ½ cup fat-free or low-fat cottage cheese

Dinner

tossed green salad with fat-free dressing
Asian Stir-Fry Vegetables with skinless Chicken or Tofu*
⅓ cup cooked brown rice
mineral water with lime or decaffeinated herbal or green tea

*Recipe is provided. See pages 114–115.

Dessert

½ cup fresh or frozen unsweetened blueberries

Day 3

Breakfast

1 poached egg or ½ cup Steamed Tofu*
2 slices multigrain whole-grain toast with sugar-free fruit
   jam
½ cup fresh or frozen unsweetened strawberries
decaffeinated coffee or caffeine-free herbal or green tea

Midmorning Snack

1 medium apple
4 macadamia nuts

Lunch

fresh fruit platter (a wide variety of colorful fruits) with ½
   cup nonfat or low-fat cottage cheese or ½ cup fat-free,
   sugar-free plain yogurt or soy yogurt
iced caffeine-free herbal or green tea or mineral water with
   lime

Midafternoon Snack

Murad Cellulite Solution Smoothie
carrot and celery sticks

Dinner

vegetable salad with extra-virgin Olive Oil and Red Wine
   Vinegar Dressing*

*Recipe is provided. See pages 116–117.

4 ounces grilled tilapia or tofu with Tomato Salsa*
⅓ cup cooked brown rice pilaf
steamed asparagus with lemon juice
mineral water with lime or caffeine-free herbal or green tea

Dessert

fresh fruit cup with mint

Day 4

Breakfast

½ cup multigrain hot cereal with ½ medium banana slices
   and 1 tablespoon dried goji berries or raisins and fat-free
   milk or soy milk
1 medium orange
decaffeinated coffee or caffeine-free herbal or green tea

Midmorning Snack

1 small pear
4 walnuts

Lunch

1 cup vegetable soup
4 ounces canned water-packed tuna or 1 cup garbanzo beans
   with tomato and onion slices
carrot sticks
2–5 low-fat whole-grain crackers
1 nectarine
1 cup tomato or vegetable juice

*Recipe is provided. See page 117.

Midafternoon Snack

Murad Cellulite Solution Smoothie

Dinner

tossed green salad sprinkled with 1 tablespoon dried goji berries or dried cranberries with fat-free dressing

baked skinless chicken or turkey breast or vegetarian soy "chicken" patty

1 cup steamed mixed vegetables with lemon and herb seasoning

1 slice whole wheat bread lightly brushed with flaxseed oil and sprinkled with garlic salt

mineral water with lime or caffeine-free herbal or green tea

Dessert

fresh fruit smoothie (blend your favorite fresh fruits with 1 cup soy milk and crushed ice)

Day 5

Breakfast

1 whole wheat English muffin topped with 2 tablespoons natural-style almond or peanut butter and ½ medium banana slices

½ cup fresh or unsweetened frozen blueberries

decaffeinated coffee or caffeine-free herbal or green tea

Midmorning Snack

Murad Cellulite Solution Smoothie
½ cup raw vegetables

Lunch

tossed green salad with extra-virgin olive oil and lemon juice
1 cup Vegetarian Split Pea with Barley Soup*
2–5 low-fat whole-grain crackers
1 medium orange
iced caffeine-free herbal or green tea or mineral water with
    lime

Midafternoon Snack

1 cup vegetable juice cocktail
carrot and celery sticks

Dinner

1 medium tomato, sliced, with fat-free red wine dressing
Chicken and Black Bean Burrito* or Vegetarian Black Bean
    and Vegetable Burrito* prepared with whole wheat tor-
    tilla and Tomato Salsa*
steamed broccoli with lemon
sparkling mineral water with lime or caffeine-free green tea

Dessert

1 slice or 1 cup cubed watermelon

Day 6

Breakfast

½ medium grapefruit
½ cup low-fat granola cereal with fat-free milk or soy milk
decaffeinated coffee or caffeine-free herbal or green tea

*Recipe is provided. See pages 113 and 117–118.

Midafternoon Snack

4 walnuts
2 tablespoons dried goji berries or raisins

Lunch

Murad Cellulite Solution Smoothie
large vegetable salad topped with ½ cup cubed tofu with fat-
   free herbal dressing
2–5 low-fat whole-grain crackers

Midafternoon Snack

1 cup tomato or vegetable juice cocktail
2 Scandinavian-type whole-grain rye crackers

Dinner

1 cup minestrone soup
4 ounces broiled salmon or 1 cup Vegetarian Chili*
⅓ cup cooked brown rice
steamed fresh green beans
mineral water with lime or caffeine-free herbal or green tea

Dessert

½ cup mixed fresh fruit topped with ¼ cup plain or fruit-
   flavored fat-free, sugar-free yogurt or soy yogurt and 1
   tablespoon dried goji berries, raisins, or dried cranberries

*Recipe is provided. See page 119.

Day 7

Breakfast

Murad Cellulite Solution Smoothie
whole-grain waffle topped with ½ cup unsweetened apple-
    sauce, sprinkle of cinnamon, and 1 teaspoon chopped
    walnuts
decaffeinated coffee or caffeine-free herbal tea

Midmorning Snack

1 cup vegetable juice
carrot and celery sticks

Lunch

vegetable soup
Veggie Sandwich on Whole Wheat Pita* with chicken,
    salmon, or Hummus*
1 medium orange
iced caffeine-free herbal or green tea or mineral water with
    lemon

Midafternoon Snack

1 medium apple
2 cups air-popped popcorn

Dinner

vegetable salad with Olive Oil and Lemon Juice Dressing*
1 cup cooked whole wheat pasta topped with 1 cup steamed
    mixed vegetables (broccoli and cauliflower florets, carrot
    and zucchini slices) and 2 ounces cooked skinless white

*Recipe is provided. See pages 119–120 and 114.

meat chicken (cut into cubes), or ½ cup baked and cubed
tofu, all covered with ½ cup low-fat marinara sauce
iced caffeine-free herbal or green tea

Dessert

tropical protein smoothie (1 cup pineapple juice, ½ banana,
1 scoop soy protein isolate powder, crushed ice)

Murad Cellulite Solution Smoothie

½ cup pomegranate juice (unsweetened)
½ cup soy milk
½ cup blueberries (fresh or unsweetened frozen)
1 tablespoon lecithin granules
1 tablespoon ground flaxseed
2 tablespoons dried goji berries (if available)
3 to 4 ice cubes or crushed ice (optional)
Splenda (sucralose) or Stevia extract (optional)

Place all ingredients in a blender and liquefy.

Fat-Free Oriental Dressing

¼ cup soy sauce or Bragg Liquid Aminos
¼ cup rice vinegar
¼ cup water
¼ teaspoon minced fresh gingerroot
¼ teaspoon minced garlic

1 teaspoon Splenda (sucralose) or Stevia extract powder, as
   or if needed

Combine all the ingredients in a blender and blend until smooth.
Makes ¾ cup.

Fat-Free Vinaigrette Dressing

3 tablespoons fat-free plain yogurt or soy yogurt
3 tablespoons chopped fresh cilantro
2 tablespoons lemon juice
2 tablespoons lime juice
2 tablespoons raspberry vinegar
2 tablespoons water
1 tablespoon Splenda (sucralose) or Stevia extract powder,
   as or if needed
1 teaspoon chili powder
½ teaspoon onion powder
½ teaspoon ground cumin

Combine all the ingredients in a blender and blend until smooth.
Makes ¾ cup.

Flax-Goji Golden Citrus Dressing

This flavorful dressing is great on salads and raw veggies. It is also
delicious as a topping to lightly steamed vegetables. It provides
omega-3 fatty acids, antioxidants, and B vitamins.

½ cup flaxseed oil
½ cup water

¼ cup fresh lemon juice
¼ cup fresh orange juice
¼ cup dried goji berries (or dried cranberries)
3 tablespoons nutritional yeast flakes
2 tablespoons Bragg Liquid Aminos or tamari soy sauce
1 tablespoon apple cider vinegar

Combine all the ingredients in a blender and blend until smooth. Store dressing in a well-sealed jar in the refrigerator for up to two weeks. *Makes 2 cups.*

Chicken-Vegetable Soup

2 cups vegetable broth
1 cup fresh or frozen corn kernels
1 celery stalk, diced
1 small carrot, diced
1 small onion, diced
1 cup cooked skinless, boneless chicken breast, diced or shredded
½ cup tomatoes, diced
2 tablespoons fresh parsley, finely chopped
salt and pepper to taste

1. In a saucepan, combine the vegetable broth, corn, celery, carrot, and onion. Bring to a boil.
2. Reduce the heat, cover, and simmer for 25–30 minutes or until the vegetables are tender.
3. Stir in the chicken, tomatoes, parsley, and salt and pepper. Heat thoroughly. *Makes 6 servings.*

Vegetarian Split Pea with Barley Soup

1 cup split peas, rinsed and drained
2 carrots, diced
2 stalks celery, diced
1 medium onion, minced
6 cups water or vegetable broth
¼ cup barley, rinsed and drained
1 bay leaf
¾ teaspoon sea salt
⅛ teaspoon white pepper
⅛ teaspoon dried parsley
⅛ teaspoon dried thyme
1 clove garlic, minced
½ tablespoon lemon juice
1 tablespoon extra-virgin olive oil
chopped scallions, for garnish

1. In a large soup pot, combine the split peas, carrots, celery, onions, and water or broth. Bring to a boil. Stir in the barley, bay leaf, sea salt, pepper, parsley, thyme, garlic, lemon juice, and olive oil. Reduce the heat and simmer, partly covered, for 1½–2 hours. Occasionally stir as needed. Add additional salt and pepper to taste if desired.
2. When the soup has become thick, turn off the heat. Cover and let it sit for 15 minutes. Discard the bay leaf. Stir. Garnish with chopped scallions. *Makes 6 servings.*

Olive Oil and Lemon Juice Dressing

3 tablespoons extra-virgin olive oil
1 tablespoon fresh lemon juice
½ small clove garlic, finely minced
1 teaspoon sea salt

In a small bowl, mix all the ingredients vigorously with a wire whisk. *Makes about ¼ cup, enough for 4 salads.*

Steamed Vegetables with Low-Fat Marinara Sauce

2 cups broccoli florets
2 cups cauliflower florets
2 medium carrots, diagonally cut
1 cup string beans, diagonally cut
2 medium zucchini, cut into ¼-inch rounds
2 medium green, red, or yellow bell peppers (or a
    combination), cut into 1-inch strips
1½ cups low-fat marinara sauce, heated

1. In a pot of boiling water, lightly steam the vegetables in a steamer basket until they are cooked but still crunchy.
2. Arrange the vegetables on a platter. Top with low-fat marinara sauce. *Makes 4 servings.*

Asian Stir-Fry Vegetables with Chicken or Tofu

Vegetable Stir-Fry
1½ tablespoons soy sauce or Bragg Liquid Aminos

¼ cup vegetable broth or water
2 teaspoons canola oil
2 teaspoons minced garlic
1 teaspoon minced fresh ginger
1 large carrot, diagonally sliced in very thin strips
1 cup celery, diagonally sliced in small pieces
1 cup snow peas, stems and strings removed
2 medium red bell peppers, cut into 1-inch strips
1 cup sliced shiitake mushrooms
½ cup scallions, diagonally sliced
     (including green tops)

1. Combine the soy sauce or Bragg Liquid Aminos, vegetable broth or water, and canola oil.
2. Heat a nonstick wok or skillet over high heat and add the soy sauce mixture. Add the garlic, ginger, carrot, celery, snow peas, peppers, mushrooms, and scallions. Stir constantly while cooking over high heat for about 2 minutes. Add small amounts of additional water if needed. The vegetables should be tender and crisp.
3. Add the chicken or tofu and blend thoroughly. Cook until desired temperature and texture. Serve with brown rice. *Makes 4 servings.*

Prepared with Chicken
2 teaspoons tamari soy sauce or Bragg Liquid Aminos
2 teaspoons rice vinegar
½ teaspoon minced fresh ginger
½ teaspoon minced garlic
2 tablespoons vegetable broth
4 cooked boneless, skinless chicken breast halves, fat trimmed and cut into ½-inch strips

1. In a bowl, combine the tamari or Bragg Liquid Aminos, vinegar, ginger, garlic, and vegetable broth.
2. Add the chicken pieces and toss together. Cover the bowl and refrigerate for about ½ hour.
3. Add the chicken mixture to the wok and stir-fry.

Prepared with Tofu
¼ cup tamari soy sauce or Bragg Liquid Aminos
½ teaspoon minced fresh ginger
½ teaspoon minced garlic
1 package (14 ounces) firm tofu, well drained and cut into
    ½-inch cubes

1. Preheat the oven to 350°F. In a bowl, whisk together the soy sauce or Bragg Liquid Aminos, ginger, and garlic.
2. Add the tofu and gently stir to coat each cube.
3. Spread the tofu on an oiled baking sheet and bake for a few minutes, until the tofu is hot and golden on the outside. With a spatula, you may need to move the cubes around on the baking sheet to heat evenly while baking.
4. Add the tofu to the wok and stir-fry.

Steamed Tofu

½ cup firm tofu, cut into ½-inch cubes
4 tablespoons tamari soy sauce or Bragg Liquid Aminos
¼ teaspoon minced ginger

1. In a steamer, lightly steam the cubed tofu for 5 minutes.
2. Flavor with a mixture of soy sauce and minced ginger. Or you can use any fat-free flavorful sauce.

Olive Oil and Red Wine Vinegar Dressing

4 tablespoons extra-virgin olive oil
½ cup red wine vinegar
3 cloves fresh garlic, minced
⅛ teaspoon dried oregano
⅛ teaspoon dried thyme

Place all the ingredients in a glass container with a lid. Cover and shake vigorously. *Makes ¾-cup.*

Tomato Salsa

2 cups chopped tomatoes
⅓ cup chopped onions
1 4-ounce can chopped green chilies
¼ cup finely chopped fresh cilantro
2 tablespoons fresh lime juice
¼ teaspoon sea salt
Tabasco sauce to taste

Place all the ingredients in a large mixing bowl and blend thoroughly.

Chicken and Black Bean Burrito

4 ounces cooked chicken chunks
½ cup cooked black beans
¼ cup steamed fresh or frozen corn kernels, broccoli
   florets, and ½-inch diced carrots or other favorite
   vegetables
1 low-fat whole wheat tortilla
½ cup Tomato Salsa (recipe on page 117)

1. Combine the chicken, beans, and vegetables.
2. Place the mixture on the tortilla.
3. Wrap the tortilla to form a burrito.
4. Top with Tomato Salsa. *Makes 1 serving.*

Vegetarian Black Bean and Vegetable Burrito

1 cup cooked black beans
½ cup steamed fresh or frozen corn kernels, broccoli
   florets, and ½-inch diced carrots or other favorite
   vegetables
1 low-fat whole wheat tortilla
½ cup Tomato Salsa (recipe on page 117)

1. Combine the beans and vegetables.
2. Place the mixture on the tortilla.
3. Wrap the tortilla to form a burrito.
4. Top with Tomato Salsa. *Makes 1 serving.*

Vegetarian Chili

1 pound tofu, crumbled
1 tablespoon soy sauce or Bragg Liquid Aminos
1 medium onion, chopped
½ green pepper, chopped
2 cloves garlic, minced
2 tablespoons canola oil
2 cups cooked pinto beans
1 can (16 ounces) tomato sauce
1 cup vegetable stock
1 tablespoon chili powder

1. Stir together the tofu and soy sauce in a large bowl.
2. In a large pan, sauté the onion, green pepper, and garlic. Add the tofu and continue cooking until the tofu is browned.
3. Add the beans, tomato sauce, vegetable stock, and chili powder. Mix thoroughly. Bring to a boil. *Makes eight 1-cup servings.*

Veggie Sandwich on Whole Wheat Pita

You can add 3 ounces of cooked, cubed chicken breast or cooked, cubed salmon to the sandwich.

tomatoes, ½-inch diced
red onion, ½-inch diced
black olives, chopped
whole wheat pita, cut in half to form two pockets
2 lettuce leaves
¼ cup Hummus (recipe on page 120)

1. Mix together the tomato, onion, and olives.
2. Place a lettuce leaf in each pocket. Stuff the pockets with the vegetables and Hummus. *Makes 1 serving.*

Hummus

2 cups cooked or canned garbanzos (chickpeas)
⅓ cup fresh lemon juice
¼ cup tahini
2 cloves garlic
2 teaspoons extra-virgin olive oil
1 teaspoon salt
½ teaspoon onion powder
¼ cup water
fresh parsley, chopped (for garnish)

Combine all the ingredients in a blender and blend until very smooth. Add additional water if necessary. Garnish with chopped parsley. *Makes four ½-cup servings.*

Murad Food Pyramid

In the early 1990s, the U.S. Department of Agriculture revised the long-standing traditional four basic food groups (meat, dairy, grains, fruits and vegetables) into a more balanced and healthy food guide pyramid.

I have updated that pyramid for cellulite elimination and youth building. My pyramid gives you a general idea of what foods you should eat, as well as relative quantities, to provide smooth, dimple-free thighs, better hydration, firm, youthful tissues all over your body, and overall good health and wellness. It is based on my water principle.

Unlike the traditional food guide pyramid, my pyramid does not contain red meat and other high-saturated fat meat products in the protein group, whole-fat dairy products in the protein group, refined grains and carbohydrates in the grain group, or

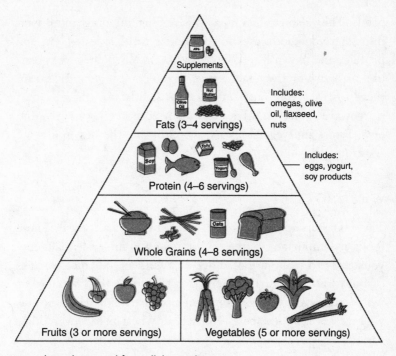

Murad Food Pyramid for Cellulite Reduction

high-calorie refined sugars or unhealthy fats and oils. I am not saying that you can never eat a hamburger, a hunk of Camembert, or chocolate. But as much as you can, substitute healthier cellulite-fighting alternatives. The more you follow the pyramid, the more successful you will be.

Fruits and Vegetables

The base of the pyramid—and the basis of your diet—is fruits and vegetables. You should eat more of these foods than any other: 3 or more servings a day of fruits and 5+ servings of vegetables. They are rich in the healing antioxidants your body needs. They also contain many of the trace minerals and B vitamins that your body uses to metabolize carbohydrates, fat, and protein, and to synthesize DNA and new cells. Whenever possible, eat fruits and vegetables raw. If you cook vegetables, steam them to retain the nutrients, or else lightly boil them. Don't microwave—that removes more than 90 percent of the nutrients. Fruits and vegetables are also probably the best source of water for your body.

Whole Grains

The next step up contains rice, pasta, bread, and cereal. These foods are important sources of vitamins and minerals that allow your body to make use of other nutrients in your diet, such as carbohydrates, fat, and protein. You should eat 4–8 servings of whole grains a day. Choose brown rice instead of white rice, as well as whole wheat pasta and whole wheat bread over other varieties.

Protein

Protein-rich foods—including omega-3-rich fish, white meat chicken, eggs, soy foods, fat-free and low-fat diary products, and beans—provide most of our amino acids. These give your body all the raw materials it needs to build collagen and elastin, the two substances necessary for keeping your dermis and blood vessels firm, strong, and smooth. Eat 4–6 servings a day.

Fats

Everyone needs fat in their diet, just not as much as most people eat and not the kinds most people eat. Limit yourself to 3–4 servings a day. "Healthy" fats are unsaturated, such as omega-3,

-6, and -9 fatty acids, flaxseed oil, extra-virgin olive oil, canola oil, natural-style nut butters, and nuts. These "good" fats keep your body hydrated, supple, youthful, and healthy.

Supplements

At the top of the pyramid are supplements. These are pure forms of the nutrients your body needs for smooth skin. Often our diets do not provide enough antioxidants, anti-inflammatories, glucosamine, lecithin, essential fatty acids, B vitamins, and trace minerals. Taking supplements every day containing these cellulite busters is the most important step in eliminating imperfections in your skin.

How Much Is a Serving?

The following guide to serving sizes will help you in your menu and meal planning.

Food Group	1 Serving
Vegetables (5 or more servings daily)	½ cup chopped raw vegetables
	½ cup cooked vegetables
	½ cup vegetable juice
	1 cup raw vegetables (broccoli, cauliflower, etc.)
	1 cup leafy raw vegetables (salad greens, spinach, cabbage, etc.)
	1 medium cucumber
	1 medium pepper
	1 medium tomato
	½ medium baked potato

Food Group	1 Serving
Fruits (3 or more servings daily)	1 small to medium whole fruit (apple, orange, banana) 1 cup berries ½ cup fresh fruit (e.g., melon cubes, grapes) ½ cup unsweetened fruit juice ¼ cup dried fruit 2 tablespoons raisins or dried goji berries
Whole grains (4–8 servings daily)	1 slice whole-grain bread 1 small whole-grain roll 1 corn tortilla 1 six-inch whole wheat tortilla ½ whole-grain English muffin ½ whole-grain bagel ½ six-inch whole-grain pita 2–5 low-fat whole wheat crackers 2 Scandinavian-type whole-grain rye crackers ½ cup cooked or dry cereal ½ cup cooked whole-grain pasta ½ cup cooked bulgur ⅓ cup cooked brown rice 1 biscuit or ½ cup spoon-sized Shredded Wheat 3 cups air-popped popcorn 3 tablespoons wheat germ
Protein (4–6 servings daily)	½ cup cooked beans, peas, lentils ½ cup tofu 1 cup fat-free milk or calcium-fortified soy milk 3 ounces fish 3 ounces poultry (skinless, white meat) 3 ounces (or one serving, as indicated on package) soy burger or soy vegetarian meat substitute

Food Group	1 Serving
	1 medium egg
	½ cup low-fat or 1 percent fat cottage cheese
	1 ounce low-fat cheese or soy cheese
Fats (3–4 servings daily)	1 teaspoon oil (extra-virgin olive oil, canola oil)
	1 teaspoon flaxseed oil (not to be used in cooking; use on salads and baked potatoes, sprinkled on foods)
	1 tablespoon ground flaxseed (use in recipes and sprinkled on foods)
	Nuts:
	6 almonds, cashews, mixed nuts
	10 peanuts
	4 halves walnuts or pecans
	4 macadamia nuts
	1½ teaspoons natural-style nut butter (peanut butter, almond butter, cashew butter)
	1 tablespoon sesame, sunflower, or pumpkin seeds

Supplements to Take Daily

- multivitamin and mineral supplement. Select a comprehensive and balanced formula containing all the major vitamins, minerals, and trace minerals; select an iron-free formula if you are postmenopausal.
- antioxidant supplement formula
- high-potency B complex supplement providing all eight essential B vitamins: thiamine (B_1), riboflavin (B_2), niacin (B_3), pantothenic acid (B_5), pyridoxine (B_6), folic acid, cyanocobalamin (B_{12}), biotin

- essential fatty acid supplement providing omega-3 fatty acids. This may be in the form of fish oil, flaxseed oil, or ground flaxseeds added to food, or in capsule form. Vegetarians or those not eating fish or taking fish oil supplements should add a micro-algae-derived DHA supplement.
- lecithin supplement. Use soy lecithin granules sprinkled on or added to foods or a liquid soy lecithin in capsule form.
- glucosamine
- calcium supplement for bone health. Most women should take 1000 to 1500 mg of calcium with vitamin D daily, depending on your dietary intake of calcium.

You can find all of these formulas separately. However, some supplement formulas, such as the Murad Firm and Tone Dietary Supplement, contain virtually all the nutrients you need in one easy-to-take package.

Six

———◆———

The Cellulite Solution Program:
Eight Weeks to Smoother Skin

You are now ready to embark on my definitive plan for a smooth lower half. If you are overweight, shedding excess fat will certainly assist in your goal to reduce your cellulite, but it is not a requirement of this program. This plan reduces cellulite through proper skin care, emotional tranquillity, and the right nutrients. By achieving these three things, you are guaranteed to look better and feel better.

When patients come to my office, I ask them a series of simple questions to determine how much cellulite and stretch marks influence their lives and their level of dedication to improving their bodies. Unfortunately, I can't see you all personally and directly evaluate your individual problem, but taking the following self-quiz on your own and articulating the degree to which your cellulite affects you will give you an honest understanding of how much your dimples have actually impacted your life and the strength of your desire to fix the condition. When taking this quiz, be honest. The more you listen to your body, the more you can help it.

Love Your Body Quiz

Please check each box that applies to you.

How bad is your cellulite?
- ❏ I have some cellulite
- ❏ It appears only when I squeeze my thighs
- ❏ I see dimpling all the time
- ❏ It is very visible on thighs, hips, buttocks, etc.

How do you feel about having cellulite?
- ❏ It doesn't bother me a lot
- ❏ It doesn't preoccupy me, but I wish it wasn't there
- ❏ It makes me feel unattractive
- ❏ It causes me to be extremely self-conscious about my looks

How uncomfortable, tender, or painful is your cellulite or stretch marks?
- ❏ Not at all
- ❏ Somewhat uncomfortable some of the time
- ❏ Somewhat uncomfortable all the time
- ❏ Very uncomfortable all the time

How embarrassed or self-conscious are you because of your dimples or stretch marks?
- ❏ Sometimes it bothers me
- ❏ It depends who I am with

❑ I think about it whenever it is exposed
❑ It bothers me all of the time

How much does your cellulite influence how you dress or what you wear?
❑ It doesn't
❑ I am always conscious of the way my body looks in clothes, especially my buttocks and legs
❑ I rarely wear short skirts and sometimes wear long pants even when it is hot
❑ I no longer wear clothes that expose my cellulite

How dedicated are you to improving your body image?
❑ Not very
❑ I am willing to test out a new program, but I am skeptical
❑ I am ready to try something new that may help
❑ I will do whatever it takes to get rid of my cellulite and stretch marks

How many treatments have you tried before?
❑ This is my first
❑ One other
❑ One to five
❑ More than five

What actions would you consider taking to reduce your cellulite or stretch marks?
❑ Just quick-fix products
❑ Just topical remedies
❑ Revamping my diet and lifestyle
❑ Commiting to a series of professional salon or spa treatments

How much does your cellulite or stretch marks stop you from participating in any sports or other activities such as jogging, swimming, or going to the beach?

❑ Not at all
❑ I participate in fewer activities than I would otherwise
❑ I wouldn't be caught dead in a bathing suit or shorts
❑ I no longer engage in any activities that expose or aggravate my cellulite

How much does the appearance of your body create issues between you and your partner?

❑ Not at all
❑ It is rarely an issue
❑ It is definitely a concern
❑ It has created a big problem in the relationship

How much does the way you feel about your body affect your sex life?

❑ It doesn't
❑ I feel very self-conscious and more inhibited because of my dimples
❑ I will make love only in the dark
❑ My cellulite prevents me from enjoying myself with a partner

Which is the most important benefit you hope to achieve from my Cellulite Solution Program?

❑ Softer, hydrated skin
❑ Improved skin texture and tone
❑ Smoothed out thighs, buttocks, hips
❑ A slimmer silhouette

Assess Your Cellulite

To simplify the process of evaluating your own cellulite, I have devised a scale to determine the severity of your dimpling on each area, from "no visible cellulite" to "extremely visible cellulite with deep dimpling and pain." By grading your cellulite at the outset, and examining the degree of your condition, you will be able to customize the program to suit your body.

Use these grades to evaluate the level of cellulite symptoms before beginning the program and again after treatment. Note that it is possible to have a different rating on the different parts of your body. For example, you may have a grade 1 on your hips and a grade 2 on your thighs.

1 = cellulite only when squeezed
2 = slight dimpling visible on skin surface
3 = advanced dimpling and skin depressions
4 = pronounced dimpling and depressed striations
5 = extremely visible cellulite with deep dimpling and pain

Think of my cellulite solution as a progressive program. As such, the effects are cumulative. I designed it as a comprehensive approach that will continue improving your skin's firmness for as long as you stick with it. I incorporated slight variations from week to week to increase the beneficial effects of the supplementation and topical therapies, and to speed up the process. The real beauty of this method is that it is flexible, allowing each individual to tailor it to her own body and her own lifestyle. It's a simple, realistic, go-at-your-own pace six-step plan.

Cellulite Solution Program

1. Look at your diet. Substitute anti-dimple foods wherever possible.
2. Follow the supplementation guidelines.
3. Exfoliate.
4. Use topical agents twice daily.
5. Modify your lifestyle to limit stress.
6. Reduce isolation and enjoy yourself.

Week 1

Smooth Body Basics

Get Organized

- Write down your goals and visualize them.
- Think about the steps and tools that you will need to get you there.
- Examine and assess your cellulite and stretch marks.

Go Shopping

- Buy plenty of the cellulite fighting-foods described in Chapter 5. Incorporate them into your diet and cooking whenever possible.
- To ensure that you get enough of these vital nutrients, buy a supplement or supplements containing glucosamine, essential fatty acids, lecithin (and its building blocks, choline and phosphatidylcholine), antioxidants, anti-inflammatories, B vitamins, and trace minerals.

What to Use

For maximum results, follow a topical skin care regimen twice a day, in the morning and at night. When you bathe, do so immediately after a dry skin-brushing routine and immediately before using the topical creams. The topical treatments are quite simple. Think of your body care regimen in the same way you think of your facial skin care regimen. In order to have truly healthy skin anywhere on your body, you need to make sure you are not overprocessing your skin with too many treatments or cleansings.

1. Before bathing, exfoliate the affected areas with a naturally bristled dry skin brush.
2. Use a gentle moisturizing soap when you cleanse your body so as not to strip your skin of natural hydrating oils. Once or twice a week, use an exfoliating scrub while in the shower to aid exfoliation and improve blood flow to the epidermis.
   - Avoid long showers or hot baths, which can dehydrate the skin.
   - Pat yourself dry so as not to strip your skin of too much moisture.
3. Use a moisturizing, stimulating cream containing hydrating agents such as hyaluronic acid (also called sodium hyaluronate); sodium PCA; phospholipids; safflower seed oil, borage seed oil, evening primrose oil, and glycerin.

   Also look in the ingredients for occlusive agents that will prevent water loss, such as ceramides and petrolatum.

   Finally, look for the addition of key topical antioxidants to strengthen the epidermal layers of the skin, such as vitamins A, C, E, green tea extract, grape-seed extract, and pomegranate extract. Anti-inflammatory agents are an integral part of the program to reduce swelling and improve skin firmness. Look for ingredients such as zinc, licorice extract, allantoin, and aloe vera. Try to find agents that increase blood flow, such as cayenne and *Centella asiatica*.

What Supplements to Take

- Incorporate up to 200 mg of niacin to strengthen and improve blood vessels.
- Take 1200 mg of glucosamine daily to repair damage to the dermal layers of the skin structure.
- Include lecithin and EFAs in your diet and supplementation to strengthen cells.
- Antioxidants such as vitamin C, grape seed, and pomegranate, are important elements of the program.
- A B vitamin complex, including folic acid and thiamine (B_1), riboflavin (B_2), niacin (B_3), and pyridoxine (B_6), which are responsible for metabolism of amino acids and fats, is needed.
- Also include the trace minerals chromium piccolinate, iron, zinc, copper, manganese, and selenium.

Take your supplements twice a day, in the morning and at night.

If you are a vegetarian, you may want to use a soy protein isolate powder that provides the nine essential amino acids every day. You may also want to obtain your EFAs from flaxseed oil and micro-algae DHA supplements.

Remember, you can find supplements that contain several of these ingredients, limiting the number of tablets you take every day.

What to Eat

Make the time for a healthy breakfast every day, even if it's just some fresh fruit to boost your antioxidant levels.

Water is essential and can come from several sources, including food. Decaffeinated herbal teas, vegetable broth, fruit juices, and fresh fruit and vegetables count toward your daily water intake. In fact, I believe that the best sources of water are fruits and vegetables. A good clue that your body needs more hydration is dry lips.

Eat one to two eggs per week. They are an excellent natural source of protein, folic acid, vitamin A, lecithin, and vitamin B_{12}. Be sure to eat the yolk, which contains the lecithin.

Fruits and vegetables lose water and nutrients the more they are cooked. Stick with foods as close to their natural state as possible and avoid overcooking, boiling, or heating whenever you can to preserve the pure nutrients in whole foods.

With this program, I am trying to get you to eat smarter. The foods I recommend are quality calories, not empty calories. Don't deprive yourself entirely of foods you crave and really enjoy; this is not a punishment. However, it is best to watch your serving sizes of unhealthy foods.

Foods to Avoid

Protein
 high-fat red meats
 processed and smoked meats: hot dogs, sausage, bacon, cold
  cuts, etc.
 fried poultry and fish
 farmed salmon and trout
 whole-fat milk
 full-fat milk yogurt

Carbohydrates
refined white sugar
candy and other processed sweets
sodas and colas (sweetened or unsweetened)
sweetened fruit juice drinks
sweetened frozen fruits
fruit jellies and jams sweetened with sugar
dried fruits with added sugar
fried vegetables
canned vegetables (with the exception of tomato products)
refined grains: white bread, white pasta, refined cereals (cold and hot), white rice, crackers and baked goods made from white and refined flour

Fats
hydrogenated and partially hydrogenated vegetable oils (trans fats) and foods containing them: most margarines, vegetable shortening, deep-fried chips, commercial baked goods (pastries, cakes, pies, crackers, and other snack foods), fast foods
butter and lard
mayonnaise
fried foods
most cheeses
bottled salad dressings containing sugar and artificial ingredients

Foods to Eat in Moderation

Protein
gelatin
lean red meat
low-fat cheeses
whole eggs

reduced-fat milk
low-fat yogurt

Carbohydrates
wild honey
100% natural maple syrup
blackstrap molasses
unrefined sugar
100% natural fruit juice (unsweetened)
dried fruits (contain all of the calories without all of the nutrients found in whole fruits)
100% natural vegetable juice

Fats
natural peanut and nut butters
sesame tahini
nuts
flaxseed (ground), pumpkin seeds, sunflower seeds, sesame seeds
olive oil
canola oil
avocado oil
olives

Foods to Enjoy

Protein
beans, lentils, peas
soy foods: soybeans, tofu, low-fat soy meat substitutes (textured vegetable protein products—veggie burgers and other soy meat alternatives)
chicken, turkey (without skin)
fish (baked, broiled, grilled)

egg whites
soy milk (calcium fortified)
nonfat milk
plain fat-free yogurt or soy yogurt

Carbohydrates
sugar substitutes (Stevia or Splenda)
fruits (raw and fresh, unsweetened frozen):
apples
apricots
avocados
bananas
blackberries
black currants
blueberries
cantaloupe
cherries
cranberries
elderberries
figs
goji berries
grapefruit
grapes (purple, red, green)
hawthorn berries
honeydew melon
kiwi
mangoes
mulberries
nectarines
oranges
papayas
peaches
pears

pineapple
plums
pomegranates
prunes
raisins
raspberries
strawberries
tangerines
watermelon
vegetables (raw and fresh, unsweetened, frozen, lightly
    cooked):
artichokes
arugula
asparagus
beets
bok choy
broccoli
broccoli sprouts
brussels sprouts
cabbage (green and red)
carrots
cauliflower
celery
collard greens
corn
cucumbers
eggplant
garlic
ginger
green beans
jicama
kale
lettuce

mustard greens

onion (white, red, and green)

parsley

parsnips

peas

peppers (green, yellow, red)

potatoes (white, yellow, red, purple)

pumpkin

radishes

seaweed

shallots

spinach

squash (winter, butternut)

sweet potatoes/yams

taro

tomatoes

turnip greens

watercress

wax beans

zucchini

whole grains: whole-grain bread, pasta, cold cereals, oatmeal and other hot cooked grains, brown rice, crackers (low-fat varieties)

Fats

flaxseed oil (added to food or in capsules in supplement form)

soy lecithin (as granules or liquid added to food or in supplement form)

Week 2

Follow the basic Week 1 program and start layering on other aspects.

- Incorporate some of the inclusive health concepts you will read about in Chapter 7 such as aromatherapy, exercise, and relaxation.
- Do some toning exercises focused on problem areas at least once a week. (If you feel comfortable doing more, by all means go for it.)
- Once or twice a week, add a five-minute skin-brushing routine before your shower or bath for boosting circulation and exfoliation. This can be a very therapeutic and invigorating me-time treatment.

Week 3

Stick with the basic Week 2 program and add to it.

- Reduce your isolation. Get out, get moving, make an extra effort to participate in social activities. It is easier to stick with the program when you are happy and enjoying life.
- Adjust your attitude. Focus on the good things, your achievements and accomplishments, and concentrate on your newfound vitality and energy.
- Sex and touch are great body boosters, and they increase your self-esteem too. Take this opportunity to connect with your partner or someone new, and learn to love your body.

Week 4

Stick with the basic Week 3 program and add to it. At this stage, you should start experiencing an increase in the firmness of your skin.

- Add a deep massage treatment (or in an earlier week, if you prefer), both as a reward for sticking with the program and for the added therapeutic benefits. Many spas offer a massage that specifically targets cellulite, such as the Murad Firm and Tone Professional Treatment, that releases tension, stimulates blood flow, and infuses the area with vital nutrients.
- Try increasing your physical exertion by adding fifteen minutes to your exercise routine every few days.

Week 5

Stick with the basic Week 4 program and add to it.

- Go to a spa and have a vitamin C cellulite infusion massage or any other relaxing, therapeutic treatment.
- Increase your skin brushing to five times per week.

Week 6

Stick with the basic Week 5 program, with the following additions.

- Increase your skin-brushing regimen to once every day before you bathe.

- Do toning exercise focused on your problem areas three times per week.
- Make another assessment of your cellulite. Compare it with Week 1.

If you are not satisfied with your improvement thus far, take a moment to review how closely you followed the program since Week 1 to determine where you may have fallen short. It may be necessary to continue for another two weeks or longer to see a visible difference. Everyone responds at a different rate, based on your grade of cellulite and stretch marks at the outset of the program. Don't get discouraged.

By now you have figured out what aspects of the program you can stick with easily and where adjustments need to be made so you can continue to successfully smooth your skin.

Week 7

Continue the basic Week 6 program. Make sure you are taking your supplements, exercising, using topical agents twice a day, and brushing your skin.

- Increase your weekly intake of foods that were recommended in Chapter 5.
- Pinch the underside of your arm to see an improvement in firmness. Taking supplements internally affects the entire body—collagen tightens up everywhere, not only where you have imperfections.

PATIENT TESTIMONIAL

◆ ◆ ◆

Jennifer
Age: 30
Occupation: Mother/student
Areas of concern: Hips and thighs

Personal testimony: Being a mother and going to school full-time really zaps my energy. As someone who eats on the go, and overdoes it on fast food, I knew I needed vitamins, but I didn't realize how important they are. As soon as I started taking the vitamins, I noticed an improvement in my energy and overall mood. While I was focusing on the change in my hips and thighs, I couldn't help but notice how great I felt. I noticed my hip and thigh area getting smoother and firmer after the first week, and after a month, I wore shorts and actually felt I looked just as good as I felt. Something else I noticed was a change in my sensitive gums. I generally have lots of bleeding when I have a dental cleaning, but for the first time in years, my gums did not bleed. My dentist asked what I was doing differently, and this is the only change I've made.

Week 8

Enjoy your beautiful, smooth skin.

This is a lifelong program. It not only helps with cellulite, it also makes your whole body healthier.

Keep up the good work. This program continues to provide smooth skin, health, hydration, firmness, decreased body fat, and decreased wasted water the longer you stick with it. Following this routine is easy, and the results keep getting better!

Clinical Program
- daily intake of supplements to address cellulite as outlined in this book
- topical application of cellulite serum

Clinical Results
Initial visit: stage-3 cellulite
Final visit: stage-2 cellulite

Additional Clinical Observations
Water measurements:
Visit 1 Intracellular 17.8 Extracellular 14.2
Visit 2 Intracellular 18.8 Extracellular 14.6
Final Intracellular 19.2 Extracellular 14.5

% Body Fat
Visit 1: 31.6
Final visit: 26.8 (a decrease of 4.8%)

BMR (Basal Metabolic Rate, number of calories used per day at rest)
Visit 1: 1,316
Final visit: 1,414 (an increase of 98 calories burned at rest)

The Cellulite Solution

The table below outlines the program discussed above. You can use this as a general guideline—there is no need to adhere to it strictly. The idea is to build on the general program throughout the eight weeks in a way that you feel comfortable with but that also includes enough elements of the program on a weekly basis to enable you to see the desired results.

8 WEEKS TO A SMOOTHER SHAPE

	Do	Eat	Take	Enjoy
Week 1	go shopping use topical cream 2x per day assess cellulite	recommended foods	recommended supplements	deep breathing stress reduction
Week 2	topical cream 2x per day skin brushing 2x per week exercise at least 1x per week	recommended foods	recommended supplements	relaxation inclusive health
Week 3	topical cream 2x per day skin brushing 3x per week	recommended foods	recommended supplements	social activity touch
Week 4	topical cream 2x per day skin brushing 2x per week exercise	recommended foods	recommended supplements	professional spa treatment

	Do	Eat	Take	Enjoy
Week 5	topical cream 2× per day skin brushing 5× per week exercise	recommended foods	recommended supplements	vitamin C infusion treatment
Week 6	topical cream 2× per day skin brushing every day exercise 3× per week assess cellulite	recommended foods	recommended supplements	relaxation inclusive health social activity
Week 7	topical cream 2× per day skin brushing every day exercise 3× per week	recommended foods	recommended supplements	relaxation inclusive health social activity
Week 8	keep it up!	recommended foods	recommended supplements	smooth skin

◆

Seven

Inclusive Health

Where Skin Care Meets Health Care

You are now well on your way to smooth thighs. You are flooding your system with antioxidants and anti-inflammatories, and providing moisturizing, protective lotion to the affected areas to prevent damage. You have added glucosamine and lecithin to your diet to repair your damaged tissues, and essential fatty acids to refill your cell walls and attract water. You have also been eating healthy foods to give your system the tools it needs to function at its highest level. There is just one piece left to complete the puzzle of an inclusive, healthy environment for smooth skin and firm connective tissue.

All the above steps will give you a healthy internal and external environment. They will give your body the tools it needs to repair and prevent dimpled skin, and to make your whole body more youthful and vibrant at the same time. But you will still not be optimally healthy if you are not happy and satisfied with your life. If you are feeling isolated and are not involved in a community of other people, if you are stressed and not taking time out to relax, or if you are not passionate about what you do, your body will not have the resiliency that it is capable of. This is the final component to what I call inclusive health. Your state of mind is just as important in overcoming skin disorders as what you put into your body and what you put onto your skin.

Listen to your body.

One question that I often ask my patients is, "Who is the most important person in your life?" They often stop and think for a minute, running through their mental Rolodex of the people in their lives before deciding that it must be themselves. If you are not around, then you can't care for any of the other people in your life. It is important to respect that and give yourself the attention and care that you deserve.

You *can* have a smooth dimple-free body. You *can* have firm skin, supple cells, and strong connective tissue. You *can* hydrate and revitalize yourself from the inside out. But your skin will never be as beautiful as it can be if you don't project the inner health and beauty that begin in your mind. There is no one cause of cellulite. If you want to truly get rid of this condition, you must address *all* of the factors that lead to it.

As with other health concepts that I have pioneered over the years, scientific data is beginning to support my theory about cellulite and stretch marks.

The Mind-Skin Connection

Think back for a moment. Have you ever had breakouts at times of high stress? Maybe while studying for an exam in school, or after a traumatic experience. Does your skin look pale and sallow when you miss sleep? These are a few effects that external forces and mood can have on your skin—and on your overall health. In fact, one survey of patients in a dermatology clinic found that 40 percent of them were suffering from psychiatric symptoms along with their skin conditions.

Think of what went right, not what went wrong.

Fortunately, there is a plus side. Research is showing that positive, external forces can have significant beneficial impact on your skin and your appearance. People who have a positive state of mind, who are passionate and free from stress, and who have regular physical and social contact with others are much more likely to lead healthy, happy lives than those who are lacking these advantages. And these benefits are more than skin deep. A study done on the power of touch on the immune systems of HIV-positive men found that after one month of massage therapy, the patients' stress levels had reduced. Even more exciting was the finding that the patients receiving the massage had an increase in natural killer cells, which are the body's first line of defense in the immune system. This suggests that those patients will be less likely to fall victim to opportunistic infections such as pneumonia.

Heal your body by giving it the best environment to take care of itself.

The focus of my philosophy is that in order to heal our bodies, whether we are addressing a life-threatening illness or cellulite and stretch marks, we need to provide a total environment of health. If our minds are not relaxed, if we are stressed and isolated, our bodies will eventually be affected, and our natural ability to heal ourselves will be compromised. A total approach to health and wellness is the best way to remain healthy, youthful, and firm. This final, necessary component of health and beauty can take any number of forms, from structured treatments such as seeing a licensed masseuse or aromatherapist to simple additions to your regular routine, like joining a yoga class, becoming more passionate about work or hobbies, or getting regular exercise.

A healthy complexion is a reflection of total wellness, both inside and out. This in turn creates a healthy environment for the skin so if problems do arise, they resolve more easily. Furthermore, skin care can lead the way to overall health. Take all the necessary steps to achieve healthy skin—the right products, the proper nutrients, and positive lifestyle choices—and your whole body will be healthier.

The symbiotic relationship between the mind and body has been appreciated for centuries around the world. However, much of the medical community has been slow to embrace these beneficial alternatives and supplements to conventional medicine. That doesn't seem to be affecting patients' desires to seek out these treatments, however. One study found that in 1990,

Americans had gone to alternative medicine practices forty million more times than to conventional ones. These patients know from experience what science is now beginning to prove: A sense of wellness can be achieved by touching and being touched, experiencing pleasant senses and a relaxing environment.

Western medicine is beginning to react. Since the 1990s, scores of American medical schools have added alternative or "complementary" medicine departments to their curriculua. These departments focus on nontraditional or Eastern medical philosophies such as acupuncture and homeopathy.

◆

Take a new path.

I opened my dermatology practice in 1972. By the early 1980s I had a thriving practice in which I was performing a great number of exclusively conventional treatments. At that time, laser treatments and collagen injections were the rage. The dermatology conventions were often focused on these treatments, and a great number of my patients were interested as well. Before too long it began to bother me that in performing these treatments I was making the skin look better temporarily without doing anything to address overall health in the skin and body. I was interested in less invasive techniques that would make my patients look better by giving them a total environment for healthy skin.

When patients needed an invasive treatment, I certainly performed it if it was appropriate. But even after many of these costly procedures, their skin would look less than optimal if it didn't have optimal health. As a doctor, it is my job to provide this health to my patients and to give them the best results available. A patient may come to me complaining of wrinkled skin, telling me she wants a Botox injection. While Botox may make the skin look smoother, it is still the same aging, weak, dehydrated skin. What that patient really wants is a rejuvenated face. What she winds up with is a smooth face that still looks aged. This is likely the reason for such a high rate of depression following cosmetic surgery. Patients are discouraged that they don't truly look younger. Unless we address all of the reasons that skin ages—unless we affect the whole picture—we cannot attain truly healthy, youthful skin, even with expensive, invasive procedures. The only time you will be truly beautiful is when you look in the mirror and are satisfied with what you see.

Attractive skin resulting from health and happiness is much more beautiful than skin that is rooted in cosmetic procedures alone. That is why I created treatments that addressed general health and wellness in addition to medical procedures that addressed only symptoms. I began utilizing noninvasive techniques such as the topical application of hydroxy acids. I also brought aestheticians into my office as full-time employees, to add the healing power of touch to my patients' treatments.

Soon my patients were experiencing such impressive results from these "supplemental" treatments that many were coming to the office just to see the aestheticians. Within a short period of time, the facialists in my office couldn't handle the demand, so in 1988 I opened A Sense of Self Skincare Institute, the first medically supervised day spa. At the spa, aestheticians could train with me to provide overall wellness to clients. My philosophy was to address both health and beauty as one, and to approach the skin both scientifically and holistically.

Making NICE

In 1998, a group of doctors from Harvard University and several hospitals in the Boston area conducted a study examining the connections and interactions between the mind and the body, specifically the skin. They dubbed their findings the NICE network, which stands for neuro-immuno-cutaneous-endicrine. They found that these body systems—the nervous systems, the immune system, the skin, and the endocrine system—are intimately connected through a dialogue of shared interactive chemicals. In short, what affects one of these systems affects the others.

They studied various external forces that affect our state of mind either positively or negatively, things like massage and aromatherapy, as well as depression and isolation. What they discovered shed some scientific light on what millions of people have known for centuries: Our state of mind has a definite impact on our health and appearance.

They discovered that several hormones and neurotransmitters released inside the body have receptors in the skin. This means that a chemical released in our bodies to help us deal with panic or stress can have unintended consequences in our complexion. This helps explain why stressful life events exacerbate conditions such as psoriasis, acne, and eczema. Similar hormones are released as a result of viruses and trauma. Although the complex network of communication within the body's systems is not fully understood, it is clear that the chemicals released as a result of stress and depression have a negative impact on our health.

Have a dream so you can make a dream come true.

If hormones and neurotransmitters released into our systems as the result of stress, panic, or disease can cause inflammation that leads to the outbreak of these conditions, there is no doubt that they can cause the inflammation that leads to the breakdown of cells and connective tissue as well. As we now know, among the many unfortunate consequences of this breakdown are cellulite and stretch marks.

It is becoming more and more common to see findings published in prestigious medical journals confirming the beneficial effects of alternative treatments as well as the strong effects our state of mind can have on our physical health. For example, a study recently found that depression is linked to poor outcomes from heart and spinal surgery and increased pain after gum surgery. Even more telling is that researchers at Cornell University found that stress and sleep deprivation among women had a negative impact on the skin's barrier function and increased water loss from the skin. As we know, these are two of the primary causes of cellulite and stretch marks.

The Healing Power of Relaxation

If negative emotions and stress can cause disease and make us less healthy, surely positive mental states, life-enhancing relationships, and therapies that make us feel good can slow the inflammatory process, leaving us healthier, happier, and as beautiful as we can be.

A key component of a cellulite-fighting strategy is to take time out for yourself to relax and enjoy life. As with the right nutrients, certain types of relaxation can provide health and skin care from the inside. There are a great number of ways for you to take some healing time for yourself. For some people, taking a warm bath surrounded by aromatherapy candles is the best way to melt away tension. For others, a walk is the ideal way to clear their head. You may find that having a manicure or massage works best to calm a racing mind, or taking some time out simply to listen to relaxing music may work best for you. Try a few techniques to see what does the trick. What works for others may not be the right method for you. Once you find the right combination of techniques that make you feel relaxed and peaceful, add them to your regular routine. Ignoring your needs and allowing stress to get a foothold can thwart your efforts toward achieving good health, vitality, and beauty.

At the Murad Spa, patients have a facial for the direct benefits to their complexion as well as for the added benefits of relaxation, pampering, and the healing power of touch. Massage is another popular and effective stress fighter. Aromatherapy can also be a soothing addition to their treatments.

Aromatherapy

A great deal of scientific literature suggests that certain scents can influence mood, anxiety, immune function, and even skin health. As an essential oil is inhaled, nerves at the top of the nose carry it to the part of the brain that controls heart rate, memory, and hormone balance, among other things. Even scents so subtle that they can hardly be identified have been found to release neurochemicals. Other findings also suggest a strong connection between the brain and our sense of smell. In fact, an impaired ability to detect odor has been noted in several neuropsychiatric disorders, including Alzheimer's, schizophrenia, and depression.

Make someone smile.

Fragrances have been used as a part of medical and religious rituals for centuries all over the world. The science of aromatherapy began in France in the early 1900s. A chemist named René-Maurice Gattefossé became interested in the medical use of essential oils after he sustained a harsh burn to his arm while working in his lab. He instinctively thrust the wounded limb into the nearest liquid he could find, which happened to be a jar of the essential oil of lavender. The burn healed much more quickly than it otherwise would have and didn't leave a scar, which he had expected from such a burn. He was so intrigued by the results that he dedicated the rest of his life to the study of aromatherapy and essential oils.

Adding an aromatherapeutic component to your bath is another excellent way to experience the healing powers of scent. It is believed that when you soak in hot water with a dissolved essential oil, it can be absorbed into your body's tissues. Once it enters the body either through the skin or by inhalation, it can have a therapeutic effect, especially on inflammatory conditions and infections, both of which involve the immune system.

Healing Touch

Touch therapies are another ancient remedy that have become popular supplements to modern conventional medicine. For years people have found mental and physical peace through treatments such as acupressure, reflexology, and massage. Scientific journals are brimming with validation for these treatments.

Massage not only benefits the muscles and tissues being kneaded and stretched, but it also has been found to reduce stress, lessen depression, improve sleep patterns, and boost the immune system. Studies have even shown that providing massage therapy to cancer patients reduces the need for potentially addictive pain medication. In many of the studies, the subjects continued to feel benefits from massage months after the treatment stopped. Healing touch therapy can take many different forms, including deep-tissue massage, skin brushing, connective tissue manipulation, and reflexology. Experiment with these techniques to find a touch therapy that you can really indulge in. Even a simple chair massage can be quite beneficial. The University of Miami Medical School conducted a study on the effects of massage on office workers. A simple fifteen-minute chair massage given twice a week dramatically reduced job stress while increasing productivity and alertness at the same time.

The pace at which these alternative therapies are being studied and validated is increasing. As further light is shed on the connection among our mind, immune system, skin, and mental and physical health, sensual therapy such as touch and aromatherapy will no doubt occupy an even larger place in our arsenal of healing treatments.

Breath

Stress is an aggravating force in illness. Even when there is an organic cause to an illness, relaxation and breathing can help the body's healing system. Without realizing it, most of us take short, shallow breaths, especially during times of stress. This leads to poor circulation and adds to tension. Try to breathe deeply into your abdomen whenever you find yourself anxious or breathing shallowly. Many people find that a few minutes of deep-breathing exercises when they awaken centers them and keeps them focused throughout the day.

Smile for no reason.

A Sample Deep-Breathing Exercise

1. Wear loose clothing and lie down.
2. Exhale through the nose for as long as you can.
3. Inhale through the nose, to a count of ten, feeling your diaphragm and your abdomen rise.
4. Try to inhale enough air to fill your lungs completely.
5. Slowly exhale to a count of twenty, pushing every breath of air from your lungs.
6. Continue for two or three minutes.

Fit for Life

I am not advocating an exercise program to address a specific physical issue such as weight loss or strength training, but rather for the more general result of feeling good in order to attain an environment of inclusive, optimal health throughout your mind and body. For this reason I recommend exercises that you enjoy doing. Too often people set a goal for themselves that they are unable to attain and wind up giving up. Make your exercises enjoyable. Take up a sport, go to a yoga class, or go for a hike. If you enjoy strength training and running, by all means go for it. The main thing is to make your exercise fun, and it will work for you.

Physical fitness is another important component of inclusive health. While it is true that exercise on its own cannot get rid of cellulite, it can help in a variety of ways.

If you don't use it, you lose it. My philosophy is based on the fact that all of our systems are interrelated. A problem with the endocrine system, for example, will affect how the immune system fights off diseases. Because of this, you want your body to be as healthy as it can be in every way. When you are physically fit, all of your systems function much more fluidly, as they do not have to deal with all of the problems that come with an out-of-shape body, such as a lack of energy, increased blood pressure, and an increased risk of diabetes, to name a few.

Exercise makes you feel good. Studies have shown that regular exercise promotes relaxation, stress reduction, and healthy sleep patterns. You may have heard of a "runner's high." It is not just a myth or urban legend. Exercise actually releases endorphins, which are in effect feel-good chemicals in your brain. In fact, regular exercise is a widely prescribed method of treating depression.

Shape up your self-image. We all want a body that we are proud of, and getting rid of dimples alone won't always give you one. If you feel like you are a little out of shape, or maybe even a lot out of shape, it may be affecting your sense of self. Try doing some exercise that you enjoy at least a few times a week. The simple act of improving yourself will make you proud. And once you begin seeing the results in the mirror, you will be feeling good all over.

Smooth out imperfections. While it is true that no exercise will fix your cellulite and stretch marks, some can minimize the appearance. Dimples are much more visible when they are covering loose tissue than when they are above firm muscles. To make cellulite less visible, try doing some simple exercises that target the areas where you have cellulite:

- Lunges firm your gluteal and thigh muscles.
- Squats firm your hamstring (back of the thigh) muscles.
- Leg lifts strengthen your lower abdominal muscles and firm your belly.

To really speed up the visual results of this program, try doing exercise targeting specific problem areas three times a week.

Stress-Reducing Yoga

Yoga builds bodies that are strong, supple, and toned, rather than hard or tense. Practicing any yoga posture in a relaxing way with slow, deep breathing and letting go may relax the nervous system. Learning to relax and reduce stress through meditation may even help to reduce the risk of heart attack and stroke.

Yoga has three components:

- postures or stretches designed to lengthen, strengthen, and relax the body
- breathing exercises that help to relax and cleanse the body, promoting mental clarity and physical wellness
- philosophy that teaches the mind to relax and to eliminate chaos and distractions

The mission of yoga is to align the heart, body, mind, and spirit, which will ultimately bring a sense of inner tranquility. In fact, the movements and techniques practiced in yoga have been found to heal some of the more debilitating effects of multiple sclerosis.

Inclusive Health Treatments

With all of the attention being focused on a complete approach to wellness, there has been more of an attempt to bring conventional medicine and alternative therapies together. I knew in 1982 when I first brought an aesthetician into my practice that true health care involved a complete program for health and well-being—one that addressed not only the symptoms but also the myriad causes of our health and beauty afflictions. Later, when I opened the Murad Spa, I asked an acupuncturist and a nutritionist to join me. This inclusive health concept of addressing all of the issues involved in wellness is the only way to truly treat our health and beauty concerns.

Today, health and beauty come together as spas more frequently provide an approach that acknowledges how important beauty is to our sense of well-being. Feeling good about the way we look is as important as being fit. People who are more relaxed, more connected with others, and eating right and exercising are healthier and more attractive as a result. Inclusive health and wellness also contribute to preventing infection and inflammation that lead to aggravation of conditions such as cellulite.

Self-Care

Of course, there is more to removing stress from our lives than soaking in a fragrant bath or having a relaxing massage. If it were that simple, many of the stress-induced illnesses and afflictions that we see every day in our society would fade away. The best way to keep stress out of your life is to stop it from appearing in the first place.

Emotional self-care is just as important a factor in health and beauty as eating the right nutrients. Truly caring for yourself involves examining your life in a thorough and honest way, and making the necessary improvements. Are there issues that are continually adding stress to your life? These must be addressed if you are to attain inclusive health. A stressful life is not a healthy one. On the other hand, if you live an enjoyable life in which you take the time to appreciate beauty within yourself and the world around you, health follows. Meaningful relationships with others, taking time out to relax and refresh, and being involved in activities that you are passionate about encourage health in a way that conventional treatments alone are unable to.

One of the most common afflictions in our society is isolation. Very often, we are so wrapped up in our careers and our routines that we have too few connections with others. Most cultures around the world believe that isolation is a major cause of illness. A report in the prestigious journal *Science* reviewed sixty studies on the subject and concluded that social relationships are intimately connected to health, longevity, and recovery from disease. And people who feel a lack of community are at a higher risk of most health problems. In fact, community could be considered the world's first panacea.

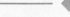

Why have a bad day when you can have a good day?

A question that I often ask my patients when they seem to be bored and isolated is, "If you had nothing to do tomorrow, what would you do?" Whatever it is, there are always others out there with the same interests looking to share them with like-minded people. If my patient says that she would read a book, I suggest that she join a book club. If she would go to an art museum, I recommend that she volunteer as a tour guide at a museum. It is this type of community activity that can give worlds of health and vitality to our internal and external lives

Interpersonal relationships and community can take many different forms. I encourage people to find something that they feel passionate about and pursue it. This may be a hobby that can be shared with others, an outdoor activity such as golf or hiking with a close friend, or a more structured approach such as a club or support group. Through pursuing your passion, you can be in touch with others who share your interests. This connection to others then evolves naturally for those who are open to it. Considering the wealth of benefits that result from positive relationships, you have nothing to lose.

There are some undesirable aspects of our lives that we have no control over. We need to be aware of these and not let them bother us to excess. It always pains me to see someone worked up and angry over a parking ticket or a business deal that went wrong, especially when it is long after the fact. While getting angry is a justifiable response to many situations, remaining angry does not help the situation. And the increased stress takes a toll not only on your ability to enjoy life but your health as well.

However, when we can change a negative situation, it is in our best interests to do so. It may be easiest to stick with a job or a relationship that is making us miserable because we are used to the routine or are afraid of an uncertain alternative. But it is well-known that stress eventually takes its toll on our health, our appearance, and our outlook on life. Beneficial life changes, although uncertain, are filled with exciting possibility.

It has become accepted that interpersonal relationships are an important part of good health. Involvement in a healing community can take on many forms, from working with a charity to spending time with a close friend. Even the time spent at the spa can be used to share your feelings with another supportive person. I believe that even when we are not ill, community activities can have a wonderful benefit to our health and sense of well-being. One thing is certain: The alternative, isolation, can be quite damaging.

At the beginning of this book I mentioned the study that was performed using the supplements I've recommended to treat cellulite. This was an independent double-blind trial, in which the subjects taking the supplements had a 78 percent increase in skin firmness in just eight weeks. That study involved only taking supplements. Imagine the incredible improvement that you will find by adding my all-inclusive approaches of topical solutions and lifestyle changes to that supplement plan.

◆

Eight

Cellulite Minimizers: Ingredients That Can Really Make a Difference

There are many cellulite remedies on the market, and even more active ingredients that make them up. It is very easy to get lost in the glut. You always hear people trying to sell you on their miracle cream with a magic new ingredient. How do you know what works and what doesn't? Is there a way to know how these ingredients are addressing your cellulite, if at all?

I have evaluated a wide array of cellulite treatments to determine their ability to alleviate the condition. I have broken them down into their component ingredients to clearly illustrate by what method these products address your cellulite and how effective they may be.

It is important to remember that until now very few if any remedies were more than simple topical treatments, which alone are not very effective in treating cellulite. You can buy many creams that contain vitamins, herbs, minerals, and antioxidants. The good ones make the skin softer, smoother, healthier, and better able to repair itself. The better creams also contain antioxidants, anti-inflammatories, and ingredients that stimulate blood flow. Cellulite-affected areas tend to be dehydrated and damaged, and need the extra benefits of moisture, protection, and increased blood supply. By increasing the moisture of the affected area. The overall appearance of the cellulite can be temporarily reduced. When you look at cellulite, you are seeing not only the dimpling effect. You are also seeing the damaged, dry skin that accompanies it and even perpetuates the condition. If you can treat this dryness and damage, the appearance of the cellulite will be minimized. However, the damage itself, and the buoyant fat cells within the skin, will remain only partially treated. As you know, to completely address cellulite and stretch marks, we need to treat them from the inside as well as the outside.

Very often, topical creams dehydrate the affected area of wasted water over several weeks or months of use. The effect of this is that the thigh that houses the cellulite does, for a brief period of time, become smaller. By association, we feel that the condition has improved as well. Have you ever heard a sales pitch for a cellulite treatment that begins, "Our product can solve cellulite by actually decreasing the diameter of your thigh by one inch!"? As you now know, the size of your body has no effect on the cellulite that is present. In actuality, while removing wasted water can temporarily decrease the size of the area treated and help to forestall future damage and exacerbation of dimpling, it does not actually repair and reverse cellulite. Also, any size that was lost will be replaced as soon as you drink water.

While topical cellulite remedies can be very beneficial, they have little effect if used alone. Creams cannot actually penetrate the dermis where much of the damage is. Creams and lotions generally reach only the epidermis, or top layer of skin. Many cellulite treatments are largely unsuccessful because they target only the external appearance of cellulite. They are unable to completely fight the damage where it lives. Now that you understand that the dimpling on the surface of the skin is merely a symptom of the underlying cause, you can see how banishing lumps and bumps requires deeper-acting treatments in addition to topical ones.

To really turn back the clock and reverse the damage, you must reach farther than just skin deep. That is where internal remedies and technology make all of the difference. I recommend going beyond simple topical remedies and utilizing science and nature's entire arsenal to combat cellulite and stretch marks. My concept of Technoceuticals includes a combination of effective topical remedies with technologically advanced treatments and formulas that can produce visible results. I incorporate nutritional supplements and a diet rich in foods that provide the essential elements to repair damage. This all-inclusive approach is the only truly effective method of treating and repairing cellulite and stretch marks.

There are nine different avenues by which cellulite and stretch marks can be effectively repaired. In this chapter I highlight each of these methods and then describe which of them various cellulite remedies are employing. Some attack cellulite through more than one of these channels, some through none. Remember, these methods work in conjunction with each other. The more of them that you employ, the more success you will have in reducing, preventing, and even eliminating your cellulite.

Nine Ways of Treating Cellulite
1. Strengthen blood vessels/increase blood flow
2. Encourage the production of connective tissue
3. Stimulate the production of collagen and elastin
4. Attract water to the cells
5. Repair cell membranes
6. Reduce wasted water

7. Prevent free-radical damage
8. Reduce inflammation
9. Promote exfoliation

Any ingredient that does not accomplish one of the nine goals cannot help your cellulite in any real way.

Treatments That Will Not Address Cellulite

While there are many products and ingredients on the market that help to prevent cellulite and repair the damage that is already present, there are also many that make strong claims but are not likely to have any effect on lumps and bumps in your skin because they do not employ one of the nine methods of treating cellulite. There are so many products on the market that it is difficult to know what will work and what likely will not. Before you spend time and money, it is always a good idea to be informed. Below you will find descriptions of a few popular products and treatments that are not likely to give you the benefit you are seeking as they do not employ any of the nine methods of treating cellulite.

Anti-Cellulite Apparel

Apparel products such as anticellulite compression hosiery are touted to create a micromassage when they are worn. Other versions include control-top panty hose that are said to reduce the appearance of cellulite while providing support to the stomach, hips, and upper thighs. One of the newest products is a panty hose brand infused with microencapsulated grapefruit seed extract to target dimpling. There are also products that offer a prosthetic top to improve the body contour line, flatten the belly, and shape and tone the buttocks by giving them a push-up effect. While these products claim to treat cellulite, compression apparel can actually have the reverse effect by constricting circulation and causing irritation.

One unique cellulite product on the market is walking shoes that are made with a patented curved and layered sole said to lengthen the body, encourage upright posture, and use neglected muscle groups. These sneakers are touted to significantly reduce cellulite and varicose veins. Unfortunately, although these products potentially have a beneficial effect on overall appearance, they will not likely repair cellulite.

Cellulite Lift

Body-lifts are generally performed on women who have lost a significant amount of weight and have been left with loose pouches of excess skin. It is the most invasive technique to restore firm, youthful contours to the body. If you look at yourself naked in the mirror and pull up the saggy skin of your hips to stretch out your upper thighs and abdominal area, you can reshape the way your body looks. Body-lifts essentially do the same thing. Lower body–lifts target the thighs, buttocks, abdomen, waist, and hips. However, body-lifts do nothing to improve the texture and quality of the skin. And while they do tighten the skin, they do not remove cellulite. The most significant drawback to this type of invasive surgery is that the scars can be extensive and the recovery is longer than most other cosmetic surgical procedures.

Cellulite Surgery

One of the problems with many of the more invasive treatments for cellulite reduction is that they tend to damage something else, especially the dermis. The only effective approach is in effect the reverse—making the dermis and vessels stronger and healthier.

Detox Diet

You often hear the claim that in order to get rid of cellulite, you have to go on a special diet to clear your body of cellulite-causing toxins. A toxin could be classified as any substance that creates irritating and/or harmful effects in the body, undermining health or stressing organ functions. Homeostasis occurs when body functions are in balance. This balance is disturbed when we take in more than we can utilize and eliminate. If our body is working well, it can handle our basic everyday exposure to toxins by neutralizing, transforming, or eliminating them. For example, many antioxidant nutrients may neutralize free-radical molecules. The liver helps transform many toxic substances into harmless agents, while the blood carries wastes to the kidneys; the liver also dumps wastes through the bile into the intestines to be eliminated. The best approach is to avoid putting toxins in your body in the first place by eating a healthy, clean, and pure diet along with appropriate supplements and lifestyle choices.

Laser Lipolisis

Laser lipolisis is a relatively new technique developed in Italy. It is performed with injections and involves the insertion of a fiber-optic laser through very small incisions that targets only the fat in the body. Amounts of 500 grams of fat can usually be absorbed and naturally excreted as waste by the body. Although laser lipolisis was not designed for high-volume applications, larger volumes of fat can be liquefied and suction-aspirated. As with liposuction, this procedure targets fat cells that are not the cause of cellulite.

Liposuction

While liposuction can change and improve your natural contours, a woman who is plagued by cellulite and undergoes liposuction to remove excess fat will be disappointed with the results, because the cellulite will still be there. Whereas liposuction can reduce fat deposits in areas resistant to diet and exercise, it is unable to affect the dermal fat that causes cellulite. In fact, in some cases it may actually make dimpling appear worse.

Muscle-Stimulation Systems

Muscle-toning systems, including ionithermie, utilize small electrical currents to provide stimulation in an attempt to tighten muscles. Treatments usually take about an hour and are done in a course of ten. There is no evidence that these systems are effective either for reducing cellulite or toning muscles. To increase firmness and tone muscles, strength training with weights, aerobics, and yoga should be the first route to take. In either case, toning muscles may make your body feel better; however, it will have little or no effect on the visible appearance of cellulite.

A Guide to Treatments That Work

Now let's take a look at the nine ways of actually preventing and repairing cellulite. It is important to remember that each method works better in conjunction with the others than as a stand-alone treatment.

Strengthen Blood Vessels/ Increase Blood Flow

You may remember that the first stage of cellulite and stretch marks is invisible to the naked eye. It is the breakdown of blood vessels. Blood vessels are the paths by which all of the nutrients essential for strength and health reach the dermis and the surface skin. While the right nutrients are incredibly important, they do no good unless they can get through to the areas that need them. Without a steady conduit for antioxidants, anti-inflammatories, water, collagen and elastin builders, etc., the skin has no way to attain reinforcements. It eventually loses the battle to cellulite and stretch marks. Utilizing ingredients that promote strong blood vessels is the first step toward smooth skin. Strong, active blood vessels can be attained through certain internal nutrients, ingredients in topical creams, as well as mechanically through methods such as skin brushing.

Encourage the Production of Connective Tissue

The second approach to cellulite treatment is to stimulate the production of the matrix (GAGs) that make up connective tissue in your body. Providing your body with an ample supply of the essential nutrients that create and restore this matrix gives you the ability to form firm, defensive connective tissue. Having a strong dermis is essential in preventing and repairing cellulite and stretch marks. As you remember from Chapter 1, it is weakened or corrupted connective tissue in your skin, more specifically damaged dermis, that allows the fat cells that form cellulite to float to the surface and become bumps and dimples.

There is another very important reason to have strong, healthy connective tissue. The primary water reservoir for your entire body, and especially your skin, is the dermis. Whenever an organ in your body needs hydration, it can extract it from your dermis, which houses extra water. A strong dermis, with ample GAGs, can help keep all of your cells, from your liver to your skin, supplied with their ideal component of water, thereby functioning at their optimal level.

Three internal ingredients are necessary to form GAGs in your body. The first and most important is glucosamine, which is the primary building block of GAGs. It is B vitamins and trace minerals that your body employs to metabolize glucosamine into GAGs. Make sure your body has an ample supply of these nutrients in order to fortify your dermis.

Stimulate the Production of Collagen and Elastin

The third method of reversing and repairing cellulite is to ensure that your body has plenty of collagen and elastin to fortify your connective tissue and keep it strong. As you know, when the dermis is strong and structurally sound, fat cells are unable to break through it and show through the surface. In order to promote the production of collagen and elastin, you need to provide your body with the raw materials for their production. The building blocks for collagen and elastin are amino acids.

Attract Water to the Cells

The fourth important component to effective cellulite treatment is making sure that all of your cells are fully hydrated. When cells do not have enough water, they are severely weakened and are unable to stand up to the pressure of fat that is fighting its way to the surface of your skin. If you rehydrate and revitalize your cells, they can become strong and firm enough to push the cellulite-forming fat cells back where they belong, below the visible layers of your skin.

Healthy, hydrated cells make up skin that feels smooth and looks beautiful. Dehydrated cells have lost their barrier ability and can no longer keep toxins out and nutrients in. This is not true just of skin cells. This applies to cells all over your body. Proper water infusion helps you look beautiful and dimple-free. It also helps you to become healthier and less susceptible to disease.

Repair Cell Membranes

If you give your body's cells the materials they need to reinforce their walls, all of your cells will have their optimal amount of water and will function at their peak level. Flush with healthy cells, the skin will be strong and youthful, and better able to keep water and absorb nutrients from other sources. At this point you may notice the cyclical nature of my cellulite solution. Every avenue of treating cellulite has its own specific benefits in dimple reduction, and each one symbiotically increases the effectiveness of all the others.

Reduce Wasted Water

Wasted water causes general problems such as bloating, weight gain, edema, and puffy eyes. It also interferes with your body's ability to repair cellulite damage. Cells and connective tissue work best in conjunction with themselves and each other. This fluid seeps in between cells and connective tissue, and in between cells and other cells, thus preventing them from properly communicating and functioning as a unit. It provides gaps that fat cells can exploit and squeeze through. There are myriad reasons, not just cellulite prevention, for removing wasted water from your system and putting it where it can be of use to your health and beauty.

Prevent Free-Radical Damage

Free-radical damage from sources such as sun exposure, smoking, and a poor diet do immeasurable damage to your tissues. Damaged skin is far more susceptible to cellulite and stretch marks than skin that has been protected from this harm. The only way to prevent and repair free-radical damage is with the use of antioxidants, both topically and internally.

Reduce Inflammation

Your body responds to damage by rushing defensive nutrients to the affected area. It does this by dilating the blood vessels and releasing specific chemicals. You notice that after an injury or infection your skin becomes warm and red. In fact, the redness that you experience from sunburn is actually the result of inflammation. While this is beneficial in the short term, prolonged inflammation actually causes the free-radical damage and cell wall deterioration that it is attempting to prevent. That is why it is important to use soothing ingredients, both topically and internally, to calm inflammation before it begins doing more harm than good. Fortunately, anti-inflammatories are widely available in a variety of products.

Promote Exfoliation

By the time we reach adulthood, our rate of cell turnover has drastically diminished, and we are left with a surface of dead skin cells that look dull and no longer provide an adequate barrier against the elements and water loss. The way to combat this is through exfoliation, the removal of surface dead cells. This can be done either chemically, using mild agents that dissolve the dead cells, or mechanically, using textured soaps or sponges and brushes that can wipe away the surface cells. When you remove cells from your skin's surface, a message is sent telling your body to create replacements. These will be strong young cells that not only look and feel healthy but also are better equipped to stand up to the onslaught of cellulite. It is important to remember that when you exfoliate, you are not so much removing cells as replacing them with stronger ones. By reducing these dead, ineffectual cells, you also increase the efficacy of topical treatments applied to the area.

Cellulite Treatments

Many of the following ingredients are essential oils and botanical extracts. Even some botanicals and antibacterial agents can cause reactions in sensitive skin types. To find out if you will have a negative reaction, do a small patch test on your forearm before using products on a large area of your body.

Aloe Vera

Aloe vera juice and oil are extracted from the aloe vera plant, which is found mainly in sunny climates. The leaves store large amounts of water. The extract improves hydration and is sooth-

ing and healing to all skin types. It is composed of water; the enzymes catalase and cellulose; minerals such as calcium, aluminum, iron, zinc, potassium, magnesium, and sodium; as well
as twenty amino acids. It is known for its healing and anti-
inflammatory properties. Aloe vera is used safely and successfully as an anti-inflammatory and as a hydrating agent both as an
edible ingredient and in topical applications.

Alpha and Beta Hydroxy Acids

The following hydroxy acids are commonly used in cosmetic
products:

- citric acid (AHA)
- glycolic acid (AHA)
- lactic acid (AHA)
- malic acid (AHA)
- salycylic acid (BHA)
- tartaric Acid (AHA)

Certain formulations of AHA products can increase cell
turnover rate and increase the thickness of the epidermis. The
effect depends on the product's pH level or measure of its acidity, the AHA concentration, the AHA vehicle cream or cleanser,
as well as how the product is used (for example, frequency and
quantity of use, where on the skin it is applied). By speeding up
exfoliation, the topical use of hydroxy acids makes skin appear
smoother. Lactic acid is commonly found in milk, pickles, and
other foods made by bacterial fermentation. Lactic acid can help
reduce the effects of photo-aging and can play an important role
in the treatment of sun-damaged skin. Glycolic and salicylic
acids are my favorite agents for increasing the cell turnover rate
and uncovering younger skin. Hydroxy acids are one of the most

popular keys to unclogging embedded cellular debris from pores and shedding the outermost layer of dead skin. Consistent exfoliation thins the dead skin that builds up, producing an ongoing vitality in skin texture and quality. If you stop using hydroxy acids, your skin will gradually revert to its normal sluggish turnover rate.

Alpha Lipoic Acid

Alpha lipoic acid (ALA) is a potent fat- and water-soluble antioxidant and anti-inflammatory. This makes it different from most other topical antioxidants, which are soluble only in either fat or water. ALA can penetrate skin cells easily through the lipid-rich cell membrane and continues to be effective once inside the cell due to its water solubility. ALA has a protective effect on vitamins E and C, thereby boosting their antioxidant abilities within the body. ALA is touted as a superior antioxidant compound. However, there is still very little data on the effects of alpha lipoic acid on human skin. Its primary function is as an anti-inflammatory. Alpha lipoic acid may be used to soften pigmented stretch marks and has been used for pigmentary disorders.

Aminophylline—See methylixanthines.

Basil

Derived from the flowering tops and leaves of the basil plant, this extract is used to relieve pain and muscular spasms, and to stimulate blood flow. It is also known for its restorative and anti-inflammatory properties.

Bioflavonoids

Bioflavonoids are a group of compounds consisting of potent plant derivatives. They have therapeutic anti-inflammatory attributes as well as strong antioxidant capabilities.

Borage Oil

Derived from the seed of borage, which grows abundantly in the Mediterranean region, Central Europe, and Asia, borage oil has an extremely high gamma linolenic acid (an essential fatty acid) content. GLA is vital for the synthesis of prostaglandin, a substance necessary for all manner of functions in the body. Borage oil has a very high content of essential unsaturated fatty acids, which are great skin conditioners and humectants that regulate the hydration of the skin. Although more study needs to be done, gamma linoleic acid may also have beneficial anti-inflammatory properties.

B Vitamins

There are eight B vitamins: folic acid, thiamine (B_1), riboflavin (B_2), niacin (B_3), pantothenic acid (B_5), pyridoxine (B_6), cobalamin (B_{12}), and biotin. The B complex group provides cumulative conditioning effects after extended and regular use. Niacin's topical form shows promise as an over-the-counter ingredient useful in anti-aging products.

One derivative of niacin, nicotinamide, has been shown to improve the ability of the epidermis to retain moisture. Topical nicotinamide was found to produce softer, smoother skin with less dryness and flakiness, as well as a reduction of fine lines. These benefits can be useful for patients with dermatitis, or dry and irritated skin. It is also useful as a treatment for aging skin, which frequently becomes dry and flaky. Niacinamide, another derivative of niacin, has been shown to be an effective skin-lightening agent. It also has anti-inflammatory properties, which makes it a potential treatment for acne and rosacea. B vitamins are beneficial in aiding metabolism of raw nutrients into new connective tissue and cell membranes.

Butcher's Broom

Butcher's broom is a plant native to the Mediterranean region. Its spines were once popular in the making of brooms, which is where it gets its unique name. Extracts from the roots of this plant seem to have the ability to strengthen and tone blood vessels, which is why it is a popular treatment for varicose veins and hemorrhoids in Europe.

Caffeine—See methylxanthines.

Carnitine (L-Carnitine)

Carnitine is a substance found naturally in the body that is used to transport fatty acids to your cells, where they are metabolized. It therefore serves the dual purpose of fat burning and cell strengthening.

Cat's-Claw

Cat's-claw is a large vine native to South and Central America. It gets its name from hooked thorns resembling claws that grow along the vine. It has been used as an anti-inflammatory by indigenous peoples for thousands of years and has recently been used successfully to stimulate the immune systems of cancer patients. Cat's-claw is also an antioxidant and has been found to increase blood flow throughout the body by dilating blood vessels.

Cayenne

The active ingredient in cayenne is a pungent substance known as capsaicin. Capsaicin appears to alter the action of the bodily compound (called substance P) that transfers pain messages to the brain, reducing pain and inflammation by short-circuiting the pain message. Topically, it stimulates the treated area and is used to increase cell function and blood flow.

Cedarwood

This botanical is considered an antiseptic with tonic and antifungal properties. It is used to reduce oil and blemishes, as a natural astringent, as a treatment for eczema, psoriasis, inflammation, dandruff, hair loss, dry or oily hair, and to soften skin. As a lymphatic tonic, it is touted to aid in the removal of body fat and to stimulate the circulatory system.

Centella Asiatica

Also called gotu kola and tiger's herb, this is an excellent vasodilator and blood vessel strengthener. It increases blood flow, thereby allowing for better absorption of nutrients. It is also often used as a diuretic, antioxidant, and anti-inflammatory, and facilitates the actions of the antioxidants vitamins C and E in areas where there is damage. In fact, this plant got the nickname tiger's herb because injured tigers often rub against it to heal their wounds.

Coenzyme Q_{10}

Coenzyme Q_{10}, also called ubiquinone, is a powerful antioxidant. It has been shown to increase resistance to disease and to strengthen the heart. Its primary function is to create a substance known as ATP in the body's cells. ATP is vital for energy. It also has great antioxidant abilities, which work especially well in the heart and blood vessels. This dynamic substance is also showing great promise in studies of the prevention of heart disease, cancer, and AIDS. It is also capable of boosting the antioxidant effect of vitamins C and E.

Copper Peptides

A peptide is an amino acid, which is a building block for collagen and elastin. Copper is a trace mineral that helps the body convert amino acids into this connective tissue. In theory, copper peptides should be an excellent source of collagen and elastin production, but sufficient study has yet to be done on this substance.

Dimethylaminoethanol (DMAE)

Topical formulas containing DMAE have been touted for their ability to improve skin firmness and lift sagging skin.

Esculin (Horse Chestnut)

Also called escin or aescin, this nutrient is derived from the seeds of the horse chestnut tree. Esculin is an excellent anti-inflammatory. More important, it has the ability to improve blood flow by filling in microscopic holes in the blood vessels. By reinforcing these veins, esculin also prevents future damage of the circulatory system.

Essential Fatty Acids (EFAs)

Essential fatty acids are so vital that they have been referred to as vitamin F. They have amazing hydrating abilities in topical creams, and when taken internally they help to build up the cell membranes and attract water to cells. Cold-water fish and ground flaxseeds are excellent food sources of EFAs.

Everlasting

This plant is a natural anti-inflammatory that is often used in aromatherapy oils and topical treatments for all kinds of skin disorders, including cellulite and stretch marks.

Fennel

Fennel is used as both a diuretic and an anti-inflammatory in some cellulite formulations. There has been too little study on it to determine how effective it is.

Ginger

Occasionally you find ginger used in a "cellulite soap" or a stretch mark scrub. While it does have antiseptic properties, its real help regarding cellulite is its anti-inflammatory benefits.

Ginkgo Biloba

Ginkgo increases the blood flow throughout the body, expanding the reach of any nutrients in the food you eat. It is also a potent antioxidant.

Goji Berries

Goji berries are virtually every method of fighting cellulite rolled into one delicious nugget. They are an excellent source of essential fatty acids, antioxidants, and anti-inflammatories, and they contain eighteen amino acids and twenty-one trace minerals.

Grapefruit

Grapefruit oil and extract have been used for muscle fatigue, stiffness, acne, fluid retention, and skin tightening, and as an antiseptic and astringent. They have also been touted for aiding hair growth and reducing cellulite. Grapefruit increases circulation, stimulates the lymphatic system, and may help to regulate body weight with regular use. It is also a good source of the antioxidant vitamin C.

Grape Seed

Grape-seed extract has the ability to inhibit the enzymes collagenase and elastase, which break down collagen and elastin. Preventing this damage from happening in the first place is much more effective than repairing it afterward. Grape-seed extract also contains a large amount of polyphenols, an antioxidant family that is particularly active in the skin.

Green Clay

Green clay is occasionally touted as a cellulite solution. Green clay contains many of the trace minerals that your body needs to metabolize nutrients into new tissue. In theory, these minerals should be effective when applied topically as well as when taken internally, but more study needs to be done on this before we can be sure.

Guarana

The guarana plant is native to the Amazon. It is helpful in cellulite treatments because of its ability to increase blood flow by dilating blood vessels. Studies are also finding that guarana has some antioxidant activity within the body.

Ivy Extract

Ivy is a climbing plant with evergreen leaves that is widely used in bath and body products for its soothing and anti-inflammatory properties.

Juniper Berries

Juniper berries come from the plant commonly known as mistletoe. Juniper berries and extracts are high in vitamin C. They have been used to treat pain and inflammation from arthritis and varicose veins, and to increase circulation.

Lecithin

Lecithin is derived from egg yolks, soybeans, and corn, among other sources. When taken internally on a regular basis, it aids your body in repairing and strengthening its cell membranes. Topically, it has a softening and soothing effect on skin and is considered a natural antioxidant and emollient. Emollients make the skin feel softer and smoother, and reduce roughness, cracking, and irritation.

Lemongrass

Lemongrass is an ingredient in preparations to treat acne, cellulite, and other skin-related conditions. It has astringent, calmative, antiseptic, anti-infectious, and antifungal properties. It is good for the hair, face, and body. It can improve muscle tone and reduces excessive sweating and enlarged pores. Lemongrass stimulates hydration and lymphatic detoxification, strengthens connective tissue, and may tighten elastin.

Marine Extracts

Kelp derived from a marine plant, is used for its anti-inflammatory properties on the skin. It is rich in minerals and has been used to supply the thyroid gland with iodine in some instances. Kelp can also be used to hydrate the epidermis.

Nutrients in algae, such as iodine, can supposedly nourish the skin and protect elastin fibers.

Dried sea salts soften water and can be used for exfoliation. People travel from far and wide to bathe in hot springs, mineral baths, and the Dead Sea in Israel because of their unique mineral compositions. Natural mineral hot springs are also quite popular for their curative and relaxing benefits in Japan.

Methylxanthines

This is basically a family of diuretics that are often used to treat cellulite. When applied topically, these substances dehydrate the treated area. After repeated use, the area becomes smaller because of the loss of water. This decrease is only temporary—when use is discontinued, any water we ingest is reabsorbed into the area. While methylxanthines have no permanant effect on cellulite, they can temporarily minimize its appearance.

Methylxanthines include aminophylline, a synthetic diuretic; caffeine, present in kola nuts, coffee beans, tea, guarana, and more than sixty plant species; theophylline, derived from tea leaves; and theobromine, derived from the seeds of the coca plant, present in chocolate.

Mint Extract

Mint extract is occasionally used in cosmetic products for its aromatic and anti-inflammatory capabilities.

Oat Beta Glucan

Oat beta glucan is an ingredient used in topical creams. It firms the skin on contact, immediately improving the appearance of sagging or uneven skin.

Pine

Pine oil is derived from steam distillation of wood from pine trees. It has been used for its disinfectant, anti-inflammatory, and diuretic properties. It also stimulates circulation.

Pomegranate

Pomegranate is my favorite source of antioxidants. When applied topically to the skin, pomegranate extract has an effect on preventing skin cancer in laboratory mice. Pomegranate is likely the world's most prolific source of polyphenols. This is a very potent family of antioxidants that work primarily in the skin. They are found in grape seeds and green tea, but most abundantly in pomegranates. It is also very beneficial in increasing the protective abilities of sunscreens.

Retinoids (Retin-A, Retinol, Retinyl Palmitate)

Topical use of retinoids over an extended period of time has the temporary effect of thickening and strengthening the dermis, making it more difficult for cellulite to push its way through. There is some evidence that retinoids also increase blood flow to the treated area.

Sweet Clover

Sweet clover stimulates blood flow and decreases inflammation in the vascular system. The clover plant produces abundant blossoms that are used in herbal oils and extracts.

Tea (Red, White, Black, Green)

Tea comes from leaves and leaf buds of plants cultivated principally in China, Japan, Ceylon, and other Asian countries. Tea is a mild stimulant, and its tonic properties are due to the caffeine content. Topically, it is used to reduce puffiness in areas affected by cellulite. Green tea also contains polyphenols, powerful antioxidants that function primarily in the skin. It is thought that these antioxidants may be able to inhibit cancer in some cases. For example, the topical administration of green tea has been shown to result in a reduction of tumors that occurred following UVB radiation.

Trace Minerals

Zinc, manganese, copper, selenium, magnesium, boron, chromium, molybdenum, silica, and vanadium are called trace minerals because our bodies need only a very small amount of them in order to function properly. All of the trace minerals are necessary for metabolism of nutrients. Without these, we would not be able to break down and utilize antioxidants and anti-inflammatories. Neither would we be able to convert lecithin and EFAs into our cell membranes, glucosamine into connective tissue, or amino acids into collagen and elastin. Trace minerals are a vital part of any cellulite treatment as well as overall health. Zinc soothes skin and also aids in the healing of wounds, burns, and scars. In the skin, zinc promotes cell division, cell repair, and cell growth.

Vitamin C (Ascorbic Acid, Magnesium Ascorbyl Phosphate)

Vitamin C fights a three-pronged battle against cellulite and skin damage. First, it plays an important role in collagen synthesis, which has a firming effect on the skin. Vitamin C breaks down collagenase and elastinase, two naturally occurring substances in the body that attack collagen and elastin. Vitamin C is also a natural anti-inflammatory that helps in reversing some of the effects of sun damage. Finally, Vitamin C is a powerhouse antioxidant that has proved especially effective in battling free-radical damage within the skin.

Vitamin E

Vitamin E, both when applied topically and when taken internally, is a very potent fat-soluble antioxidant. This means that it can easily work its way into the fat-rich cell membranes in our bodies, protecting the cell walls from free-radical damage. Vitamin E is also an excellent hydrating and sealing agent when used in topical creams.

Anti-Dimple Treatments

Many popular treatments are purported to reduce cellulite and stretch marks. These range in invasiveness from gentle body wraps and massages to expensive surgical procedures.

What has not been measured is the impact that some of these therapies may have on your overall well-being and psyche, which is also of vital importance. For example, although lymphatic drainage may not be the definitive panacea for cottage cheese thighs, it may very well make you feel relaxed, invigorated, sleek, and sexy. This topic was discussed in detail in Chapter 7. I am a big believer in doing anything that feels good, gives you pleasure, and does you no harm. Being dimple-free and miserable is not a good trade-off. I want you to be smooth and happy with yourself too.

Body Spa Treatments

These are basically facials for your body. They can be wonderfully beneficial on many levels. For example, the Murad Spa in California (as well as many other spas around the world) offers our Firm and Tone Body Treatment. It begins with exfoliation of the problem area to help prepare it for a deep high-concentration infusion of firming, free-radical-fighting vitamin C. The procedure ends with a massage to relax your body while stimulating blood flow and metabolism. I am a firm believer that professional spa treatments are the ideal way to maximize any skin care regimen, whether your goal is to clear up acne, wrinkles, sun damage, or cellulite and stretch marks.

Body Wraps

Body wraps basically work by inducing sweating. They have a temporary diuretic effect in that they cause water loss in the body. Unfortunately, fat cells and connective tissue are not affected by sweating. Wraps work on other levels too, however. The body is usually swathed for up to an hour in herb-and seaweed-soaked cloths to increase circulation and firm the body's contours. You can expect to be wrapped from chest to toe (arms are optional) while lying on a thermal blanket to keep you warm. A technician then unwraps you and, as a final step, massages your body to further enhance circulation, sending oxygen to blocked tissues. Body wraps are not recommended for anyone who is dehydrated, so be wary if you drink excessive amounts of alcohol or caffeine. Because body wraps increase internal temperature, they are also not recommended for anyone with high blood pressure, or for pregnant women.

Seaweed, clay, and herbal wraps are exfoliating and they can improve the skin's appearance and texture. Depending on the herbs used, herbal wraps can be stimulating or soothing. The other action of body wraps is the diuretic effect of inducing sweating and temporarily reducing wasted water. However, as soon as you drink a glass or two of fluid or eat a regular meal, the fluid returns.

Body wraps can provide some localized edema loss, good exfoliation, some pampering relaxation, and the possible introduction of minerals. In theory, trace minerals should be effective when applied topically, but we need more evidence to be certain.

Deep-Tissue Massage

Deep-tissue massage consists of slow strokes to create microtears in the superficial fascia. This makes tissue longer and smoother.

The deep massage also loosens the connective tissue so that it moves more freely and no longer adheres to underlying structures. Deep massage followed by lymphatic drainage and appropriate stretching can also make the superficial fascia more flexible. The concurrent stimulation of the blood vessels can increase blood flow in the area, thereby increasing nutrition to the tissues.

Massage does not remove or decrease fat cells. It may improve the condition and appearance of the skin, reduce troublesome adhesions and scars, and increase the circulation of nutrients to tissues. When deep massage is too strong, it may also damage blood vessels, which defeats the benefits for cellulite reduction. Since areas with cellulite may already be sensitive, you can feel if too much pressure is applied. Deep massage provides relaxation and, if done properly, can stimulate the blood vessels and reduce stiffness.

A Sample Do-It-Yourself Massage

Begin by gently stroking with firm, moderate pressure, taking care not to press so hard that you break capillaries and bruise yourself. You can massage any time of the day, but it's best to wait at least two hours after eating. The most convenient time for most women is after a bath or shower—and preferably one that includes a brisk body rub with a loofah friction mitt. A bath is relaxing, and massage benefits you most when you are relaxed. Massaging areas of cellulite once or twice a day improves blood and lymph circulation and minimizes the appearance of the hard fatty lumps. Apply a moisturizing cream or oil to the area to be massaged, so that your hands can glide smoothly over the skin. Use your thumb and fingers to grip the skin and fatty layer beneath it. Then knead in small circular movements as though working with dough. Next, massage across the skin using the base of the palm of your hand, working in long, sweeping strokes toward the heart. Alternately, try a special handheld massager, which must be used with an oil or lotion to avoid excessive friction and broken capillaries.

Dermal Fillers

Fillers are an expensive and temporary method to improve the cosmetic appearance of dimpling. After a series of injections of human fat or another filling agent, the dimples may appear less obvious until the material eventually reabsorbs and the dimples return. This is a very costly and time-intensive procedure. To improve cellulite, any substance would have to be injected intradermally—into the skin and not below the skin—with a fine needle. For example, injectable hyaluronic acid gel may produce the effect of building GAGs. Injectable bovine (from cows) and human collagen may stimulate fibroblasts to strengthen the dermal layer. While these improve the appearance of uneven skin, the results wear off.

Electronic Anticellulite Devices

There are a few noninvasive, nonsurgical treatments for skin contour irregularities that are approved by the FDA for the "temporary reduction in the appearance of cellulite." One unit is a vacuum device that creates suction to temporarily immobilize and lift your fatty tissue, while dual rollers create deep, subdermal massage to the connective tissue. This stretches the connective tissue, increases blood and lymphatic flow, and exfoliates the skin.

These sessions take forty-five to ninety minutes and have been described as feeling like a rigorous massage. The typical treatment plans entail ten to twenty sessions, and once-a-month maintenance sessions, for an indefinite period of time. Once you stop having treatments, your skin texture and tone revert to their original state.

Treatments may leave you feeling invigorated, but long-term results have never been established either clinically or scientifically. These devices are also used as an adjunct to liposuction to smooth out potential imperfections that occur with large-volume fat reduction. They may cause bruising and damage to the dermis.

Iontophoresis

Iontophoresis devices are prescribed products that use electrical currents to feed mineral salts directly into your body. With the right nutrients, this method can potentially be used to treat cellulite. However, the only approved use for iontophoresis is for diagnosing cystic fibrosis.

Manual Lymphatic Drainage

The lymph system is the body's waste disposal system. It acts as a natural defense in the body by clearing away bacteria, cell debris, excess water, proteins, and wastes from the connective tissue and returning it to the bloodstream for ultimate removal by the kidneys. Many immune processes occur in the lymph nodes. If the pathways become congested, damaged, or severed, then fluids can build up in the connective tissue, leading to edema, swelling, and inflammation. If there are any abnormalities in the tissues (as the result, for example, of chronic inflammation, recent surgery, congestion), the lymphatic system transports the damaged cells, inflammatory substances, and wasted water away from the area. The quicker this happens, the faster the recovery.

Manual lymphatic drainage, the technique of gentle lymph massage, enhances and stimulates the lymphatic system to remove wastes more rapidly from around the cells and in the tissues, sending it back into the lymphatic system for removal and ultimate cleansing.

Dr. Emil Vodder developed MLD in France in the 1930s. He came up with a massage technique to stimulate the pump of the lymphatic system with gentle stationary circles on lymph nodes. MLD affects the nervous system, smoothes muscles, and increases fluid movement in the connective tissue. It involves a slow, rhythmical touch applied by the therapist in the form of a light massage that can be very relaxing. It has a calming, stress-reducing effect that can also reduce pain.

For cellulite treatment, the therapist first assesses the condition of the skin: color, texture, temperature, moisture, and elasticity. The next step is to look at the contour of the hips and legs, and hunt for skin thickening, ridges, lumps, and visible scars that run across lymph vessels and may obstruct lymph drainage. He or she examines visible veins, looking for redness, swelling, heat, and pain. Lymphatic drainage is very useful before and after cosmetic surgery to decrease bruising, edema, and inflammation. The effects are only temporary, and it has not been shown to reduce dimpling in the long term, but it may provide relaxing benefits.

Mesotherapy

Mesotherapy is microinjections of conventional or homeopathic medication and/or vitamins into the middle of the dermis, in order to deliver healing or corrective treatment to a specific area of the body. Injections of various substances, from vitamins to drugs to anesthetics, are used for many ailments and conditions, including cellulite reduction. At present, there are no substantial clinical studies to prove that this technique is a cure for cellulite. Mesotherapy is administered directly to the desired area of the body. As many as one hundred to five hundred skin-deep injections are delivered into trouble spots such as the hips or thighs. For cellulite, the injections usually include tiny amounts of the diuretic aminophylline and the heart medication isoproterenol, which is said to melt fat, along with other homeopathic substances.

The problem with mesotherapy is that there is no standardization or specific formula. The ingredients change with each practitioner of the technique, and results may vary depending on what is injected and in what ratio. The number of treatments needed depends on several factors, such as the severity of the condition and the cause of the problem. Long-term, chronic cellulite and wrinkles may require at least fifteen sessions before you notice any result.

Microdermabrasion

Microdermabrasion is a popular alternative to chemical peeling that utilizes a blast of aluminum oxide or salt crystals to exfoliate skin superficially. Microdermabrasion uses tiny particles that pass through a vacuum tube to gently scrape away the aging skin and stimulate new cell growth. Because of the superficial nature of this technique, multiple treatments are usually required. The results are similar to a light peel. There has been a proliferation of handheld devices designed to be used at home as an alternative to salon or clinical microdermabrasion treatments. Although not as effective as professional treatments, these devices do exfoliate and can be used for the body as well as the face. As an adjunctive therapy, microdermabrasion may accelerate the use of certain topical treatments such as moisturizers, antioxidants, and anti-inflammatories.

Nonablative Lasers

By pointing these lasers at the affected area, the collagen and elastin bundles become heated and move closer to the surface. This has the effect of firming the skin's dermis and evening out some imperfections. These lasers may also increase the distance between the dermis and the fat that causes cellulite. The results of this treatment are temporary.

Peels

Peels utilize a strong concentration of a chemical exfoliating agent to resurface the skin. New cells made by the remaining dermis result in a newly healed surface, and voilà—healthier and more radiant skin is uncovered. Chemical peels are flexible and can be adapted to various levels depending on how deep a peel you want and how sensitive your skin is. Glycolic acid is commonly used and is generally safer than trichloracetic acid (TCA). TCA peels can penetrate deeper into the skin to destroy and remove the outer layers. They work by actually damaging your skin to the point that your body needs to build new collagen and elastin bundles. You might feel a burning or stinging sensation, and there will be moderate swelling of the treated areas for about a week and minimal scabbing. Further healing and toughening of the new skin take place for the next few weeks following a TCA peel. While this will work in thickening and firming the dermis, the effect is temporary, and there is a risk of scarring. This risk is minimized when glycolic acid is used instead of TCA.

Skin Brushing

Skin brushing is a simple technique that stimulates blood and lymph flow, removes dead skin cells, and encourages new cell growth. You need only a loofah or a body brush with natural rather than synthetic bristles and a long handle or strap so that you can reach your back and buttocks. To work your whole body, start at your feet and work your way up. Brushing the whole body in this way takes between three and five minutes, depending on how many strokes you give to each area. Pay particular attention to the cellulite-prone areas, using small circular movements. It is best done in the morning—the resulting acceleration of blood flow can be quite invigorating. The difference in your skin may be visible after just a few sessions—it becomes very soft and develops a rosy glow. Dry skin brushing must be done gently without harsh or rigorous rubbing that can damage the dermis. Overbrushing causes the skin to turn red and become irritated.

Treatments that stimulate the blood flow to the skin can have beneficial effects when combined with the other principles of internal and external skin care. Although there are no blood vessels in the epidermis, the dermis is rich with blood vessels, and the epidermis receives nutrients and oxygen supply from the dermis. The blood vessels in the dermis are continuations of larger vessels located deeper in the body that branch out into smaller vessels as they approach the surface of the skin. Brushing can help to stimulate these vessels.

Thalassotherapy

Thalassa is the Greek word for "sea." It is well-known that seawater is rich in minerals and nutrients, including iodine, copper, zinc, iron, strontium, and plankton. Thalassotherapy combines the application of seaweed and heated seawater to dilate the pores and blood vessels, making the skin more permeable and open to the absorption of sea minerals. This method has been used to treat arthritis and other medical conditions, as well as for slimming and cellulite reduction.

Glossary

acetylcholine. A chemical neurotransmitter that is released by nerve cells.

acetyl glucosamine. A skin-conditioning ingredient in cosmetics.

acupuncture. An ancient Eastern healing technique based on Taoist philosophy. Acupuncture can be administered using needles, low-voltage electric current (electroacupuncture), or pinpoint massage (acupressure).

adipose tissue. Fat-filled tissue that supplies the body's energy.

allantoin. A botanical extract used in hand lotions and other skin-soothing formulas because of its ability to help heal wounds and to stimulate the growth of healthy tissue.

allergen. A substance that causes an allergic reaction.

algae extract (seaweed extract). An active substance used to normalize the skin's moisture content and provide suppleness and firmness to the epidermis. Benefits antioxidant function, the skin's immune defenses, dermal condition, skin restructuring, wrinkle reduction, and tissue renewal.

aloe vera. Aloe gel, derived from the thin-walled cells of the plant, is considered an effective healing ingredient for the treatment of burns and injuries. Aloe is employed for its hydrating, softening, and anti-inflammatory benefits in skin preparations.

alpha hydroxy acids (AHAs). Naturally occurring substances derived from various sources, including citrus fruits, apples, sugarcane, and sour milk. AHAs affect both the epidermis and dermis. They have been used since the days of Cleopatra for their skin-conditioning benefits.

alpha lipoic acid. A potent and versatile antioxidant.

amino acids. The body's building blocks, from which proteins are constructed. The body's collagen and elastin are made of chains of amino acids.

anticoagulant. A substance that inhibits blood clotting.

anti-inflammatory. A substance that counteracts inflammation, a response to cellular injury that is marked by redness, heat, pain, and swelling.

antioxidant. A nutrient or chemical that reacts with and neutralizes free radicals or chemicals that release free radicals. Antioxidants intercept the free radicals and prevent them from damaging molecular structures such as DNA. Also called free-radical scavenger.

arbutin. An anti-infective derived from the dried leaves of the genus *Vaccinium,* including blueberries, cranberries, bearberries, and most pear plants. Arbutin has been used to treat hyperpigmentation.

arnica (wolfsbane). A botanical credited with antiseptic, astringent, antimicrobial, anti-inflammatory, anticoagulant, circulation-stimulating, and healing properties. It may promote the removal of wastes from the skin, aids in the growth of new tissue, and is an antiallergenic.

aromatherapy. The inhalation of evaporated essential oils to effect a number of health benefits.

ascorbic acid (vitamin C). One of the most important water-soluble vitamins. Ascorbic acid is a powerful antioxidant with many benefits for the skin and body. It is necessary for healthy teeth, bones, and blood vessels. Vitamin C helps to maintain the skin's barrier function and is effective for preventing and correcting photodamage when used topically.

ascorbyl palmitate. A salt of ascorbic acid used as an antioxidant and preservative in cosmetic creams and lotions.

barrier function. The skin's ability to act as an active barrier that controls or influences such processes as moisture loss and temperature.

bath salts. Used to chemically soften bathwater and to perfume the skin. They are usually made from rock salt or sodium thiosulfate that has been sprayed with alcohol, dye, or perfume. Rock salt is common table salt and has been used for treating inflammation of the skin. Bath salts may also be used for aromatherapy.

bearberry extract. Bearberry contains a high concentration of the antiseptic arbutin. It has an anti-inflammatory effect and is also used to treat hyperpigmentation.

beta-glucans. By stimulating the formation of collagen, beta-glucans reduce the appearance of fine lines and wrinkles. Used as a thickener and as a skin conditioner.

bioflavonoid. A plant derivative with antioxidant properties and anti-inflammatory capabilities.

bladder wrack. A type of seaweed extract used to treat wounds, bruises, and swelling. It contains iodine and sulfur amino acid, which stimulate, revitalize, and nourish the skin. Has potential tissue renewal action and positive effects on facial wrinkles.

BMR. Basal metabolic rate. The number of calories burned per day at rest.

body-lift. Surgical procedure to redrape and remove excess skin of the hips, thighs, and abdomen.

borage seed oil (borage oil). An effective anti-irritant that has hydrating properties and an ability to improve dry, itchy skin.

botanicals. Cosmetic ingredients derived directly from plants.

butcher's-broom extract. A botanical that has slimming and anticellulite effects, as well as diuretic and anti-itching properties.

B vitamins. A group of eight vitamins (thiamine, riboflavin, niacin, pyridoxine, folic acid, cyanocobalamin, pantothenic acid, and biotin) essential for the metabolism of proteins, fats, and carbohydrates.

capillary. Any of the smallest blood vessels connecting arterioles with venules and forming networks throughout the body.

carbohydrates. Neutral compounds of carbon, hydrogen, and oxygen (as sugars, starches, and cellulose), most of which are formed by green plants and constitute a major class of animal foods.

cat's-claw. A tropical vine found in South America. It has many benefits, including antioxidant and anti-inflammatory.

cayenne. The active ingredient in cayenne is a pungent substance known as capsaicin, which appears to alter the action of the bodily compound (called substance P) that transmits pain messages to the brain, reducing pain and inflammation by short-circuiting the pain message. Cayenne helps to increase circulation by stimulating blood vessels, causing vasodilation.

cedarwood oil. This clear oil has antiseptic, sedative, and astringent properties. It is also valuable for use on skin eruptions and to relieve itching.

cell membrane. The outer wall of a cell that holds in water and vital elements such as the nucleus.

cellulite. The lumpy fat generally found in the thighs, hips, and buttocks of many women.

centella asiatica. This plant has been used in medicine for centuries both topically and systematically for wound healing and stimulating blood flow. Also called gotu kola and tiger's herb.

ceramides. Lipids (fats) that act primarily in the uppermost skin layer, affecting the intercellular spaces of the stratum corneum where they form a protective barrier and reduce natural transepidermal water loss.

choline. A building block of lecithin. The body uses choline to manufacture other valuable biochemicals. Choline is found in green leafy vegetables, fish, peanuts, organ meats, soybeans, yeast, and wheat germ.

clover extract. Clover produces abundant blossoms that are used in herbal oils and extracts.

collagen. A structural protein that gives the skin and other tissues strength and tone. Collagen enhances the moisture-retaining ability of topical products, contributes sheen, builds viscosity, and leaves the skin smooth and soft.

copper. Copper itself is nontoxic, but soluble copper salts, notably copper sulfite, are skin irritants. Copper plays an active role in melanin and collagen production.

cypress oil. Useful as an antiseptic, with healing, soothing, and antispasmodic properties.

dermal fillers. Injectable materials that help to replace lost soft tissue. Common fillers are collagen and hyaluronic acid.

dermis. The second layer of skin, under the epidermis. This layer is connective tissue made up of glycosaminoglycans. It contains the vast network of capillaries and blood vessels, along with collagen and elastin fibers.

diuretic. A substance that increases the excretion of sweat or urine.

echinacea. A plant whose roots and leaves are thought to be a natural antibiotic and immune enhancer. Topical applications are antiseptic and soothing to the skin.

edema. Excessive fluid buildup in body tissues.

elastin. The elastic tissue in the body that increases flexibility. Collagen and elastin are similar.

emollient. A preparation that helps make the skin feel softer and smoother and reduces roughness, cracking, and irritation. It may help retard the fine wrinkles of aging.

emulsifiers. Emulsifiers hold the oil-based and water-based ingredients together, helping stabilize their interaction.

enzymes. Proteins produced by cells that regulate the body's biochemical reactions.

epidermis. The outermost layer of the skin. The epidermis protects the skin from moisture loss, bacteria, and other environmental factors.

erythema. Excessive redness of the skin, often part of an irritant response.

esculin (horse chestnut tree extract). Stimulates blood flow, thereby promoting drainage of skin tissue and restoring firmness.

essential fatty acids (EFAs). The basic building blocks of body fats and cell membranes.

evening primrose. The oil has a high content of linoleic acid, an essential fatty acid important for the maintenance of the skin's barrier.

exfoliation. A process that encourages the shedding of superficial cells of the skin. Exfoliation may be performed manually with scrubs, brushes, or cloths, or through the application of compounds containing alpha or beta hydroxy acid.

fatty acids. The primary building blocks of lipids.

flaxseed. A source of EFAs. Flaxseed oil is important in cell hydration.

free radical. Atom, molecule, or molecular fragment with a free or unpaired electron. Free radicals are produced in many different ways, such as by normal metabolic processes, ultraviolet radiation from the sun, and nuclear radiation.

garlic extract. Garlic is sometimes externally applied in ointments and lotions to reduce hard swellings and for treating skin problems.

ginger. A plant root used mainly for its soothing and antiseptic qualities.

ginkgo extract. Credited with antioxidant properties, ginkgo also appears to aid in the production of collagen and elastin. Additionally, ginkgo is an anti-inflammatory.

glucosamine. A nutrient needed to build GAGs and help to build connective tissue.

glycosaminoglycans (GAGs). Major components of the extracellular matrix and of connective tissues. GAGs have moisturizing and firming properties.

goji berries. Berries native to China and Tibet that have high concentrations of vitamins and nutrients.

grapefruit oil. Essential oil with diuretic properties known to be a lymphatic stimulant.

green tea. Green tea contains the antioxidant flavonoid catechin. It is also an antibacterial, an anti-inflammatory, and a stimulant. In addition, it is used in sunscreens for its ability to increase the SPF.

hormones. Chemicals released from glands into the bloodstream, which affect organs or tissues elsewhere in the body.

hyaluronic acid. A natural protein and a component of GAGs. Helps absorb moisture.

hydrophillic. Describes a product that combines with or attracts water.

hydrophobic. Describes a product that repels water.

hydroquinone. Ingredient used in bleach and freckle creams and in suntan lotions.

hydrotherapy. Underwater jet massage, jet sprays, and mineral baths.

hyperpigmentation. Excess pigmentation in the skin.

hypopigmentation. Diminished pigmentation in the skin.

intrinsic aging. The natural aging that occurs regardless of external factors, also known as genetic aging.

ivy extract. A plant extract with slimming and anticellulite effects due to its ability to prevent water accumulation in the skin tissue.

juniper oil. Antiseptic, astringent, cleansing, and toning ingredient.

kelp. Seaweed used by herbalists to supply the thyroid gland with iodine and to help regulate skin texture.

keratin. A protein often used in cosmetics for its moisture retention and protective effect.

lactic acid. An alpha hydroxy acid useful for treating sun-damaged skin and as a moisturizer.

lecithin. A natural antioxidant and emollient found in all living organisms. It is an essential component of cell membranes.

licorice. A substance with skin-bleaching and soothing properties.

linoleic acid. An emulsifier that prevents roughness and dryness.

linseed oil. A yellowish oil from flaxseed that is soothing to the skin and also an essential fatty acid.

lipids. Fats, oils, and waxes that serve as building blocks for cells or as energy sources for the body.

liposuction. Surgical removal of localized fat deposits by applying suction through a small tube inserted into the body.

lymphatic drainage. A method of massage used to stimulate the contraction of lymph vessels, helping to move the lymph forward and drain wastes.

manganese. A trace element that plays a role in collagen synthesis and skin moisturizing, as a treatment for acne and sunburns.

meditation. Focusing the concentration on the breath, or on a particular thought, sound, or image for a length of time. Regular meditation results in increased energy, overall health, and powers of concentration, as well as reduced stress and anxiety.

melanin. The pigment in skin cells.

melanocyte. An epidermal cell that produces melanin.

menthol. An antiseptic, cooling, and refreshing fragrance that stimulates blood circulation.

metabolism. The chemical changes in cells that provide energy for the body.

mint oil. An aromatic helpful for scratches and insect bites. Peppermint and spearmint are the two most widely used in skin care preparations.

niacin (nicotinic acid). The active part of vitamin B_3. It is an essential nutrient that participates in many energy-yielding reactions.

niacinamide (nicotinamide). B vitamin that is the vital precursor to the body's coenzymes in ATP production. Used as a skin stimulant.

occlusives. Substances that decrease moisture loss by the skin.

olive oil. Oil extracted from olives with emollient properties.

panthenol (dexpanthenol, vitamin B complex factor, vitamin B_5). A penetrating moisturizing agent that promotes normal keratinization and healing.

pantothenic acid. A water-soluble B complex that is essential for normal physiological functions, including the body's breakdown and utilization of food.

peptide. Two or more amino acids combined with each other.

pH. The level of acidity or alkalinity of a chemical ingredient or product.

phospholipids (phosphatides). Complex fat substances that, together with protein, form the membrane of all living cells. Used topically as a moisture/emollient.

pine oil. An oil thought to increase the turnover of epidermal cells.

polyglucan (beta-glucan). A sugar molecule or polysaccharide reported to enhance the skin's natural defense mechanism. It is also credited with wound healing and promoting cellular activity.

polyphenol. An antioxidant that prevents or lessens the damaging effects of free radicals.

pomegranate. A tart thick-skinned berry that contains polyphenols.

propylene glycol (1, 2-propanediol). A widely used cosmetic ingredient and the most common moisture-carrying vehicle other than water. Used in cosmetic formula to enhance functionality.

proteins. The essential constituents of every living cell. Proteins are combinations of amino acids.

RDA. Recommended Daily Allowance, the U.S. government's suggested intake for various nutrients.

retinoid. A substance derived from vitamin A. Retinoids repair damaged skin. Retinoid treatment can inhibit the breakdown of dermal collagen and promote collagen synthesis.

rosemary extract. An herb that promotes wound healing. It also helps improve blood circulation, thereby aiding in skin regeneration.

sage. An herb used as a tonic, digestive, antiseptic, antispasmodic, and astringent.

salicylic acid. A beta hydroxy acid applied topically to treat acne by sloughing the skin.

saturated fats. Fatty acids abundant in red meat, lard, butter, hard cheeses, some vegetable oils (particularly palm oil, coconut oil, and cocoa butter), and partially hydrogenated oils.

seawater wrap. Wrap (or mask) of concentrated seawater and seaweed with ocean nutrients, minerals, rare trace elements, vitamins, and proteins. These enter the bloodstream and revitalize skin and body.

seaweed. Plants rich in minerals that hydrate the skin.

septa. A band surrounding fat cells.

spider veins. Superficial dilated vessels that lie close to the skin's surface.

Stevia. A natural, non-caloric, sweet-tasting plant used around the world for its pleasant taste, as well as for its increasingly researched potential for inhibiting fat absorption and lowering blood pressure.

stratum corneum. The outer part of the epidermis, made up of dead skin cells.

striae. Stretch marks.

subdermal. Under the skin.

thalassotherapy. Treatments using the therapeutic benefits of the sea and seawater products.

toxicity. The relative degree of being toxic or poisonous.

trace minerals. These play an important role in the proper functioning of enzyme systems, nerve conduction, and muscle function, providing the framework for tissues, and regulation of organ functions.

transepidermal water loss. The evaporation of the body's water through the skin.

trichloroacetic acid (TCA). A peeling agent that improves fine surface wrinkles, superficial blemishes, and pigment problems.

tyrosine. An amino acid used in cosmetics to help creams penetrate the skin.

ultrasound. Vibrations with frequencies above the range of human hearing.

varicose veins. Veins that are abnormally swollen and dilated.

vascular. Relating to or containing blood vessels.

vasodilator. Something that causes the blood vessels to enlarge or relax. Warm or hot water causes vasodilation and increased circulation; cold water causes vasoconstriction—the blood vessels contract quickly, which reduces circulation.

vein. A vessel that carries blood back to the heart.

vitamins. Organic substances that are essential to the nutrition of most animals.

xanthines. Compounds found in chocolate, coffee, tea, and many drugs. They act as diuretics to reduce body fluid and also dilate the heart's blood vessels.

yoga. Exercise system developed in the East using postures and controlled breathing, to stretch and tone the body, improve circulation, calm the central nervous system, and produce a meditative and whole state of being.

zinc. An important anti-inflammatory nutrient for a healthy immune system.

Acknowledgments

During the last twelve months, my son, Jeff Murad, has dedicated himself to taking my words, thoughts, and concepts and translating them into a comprehensive, inclusive health program for combating cellulite. He captured more than thirty years of dermatological experience and passionately translated my program into a book. I am so proud of him and the work he has done to help me make this book a reality.

I would also like to extend my deepest gratitude to Dr. John Westerdahl for his insight into the world of nutrition. As a registered dietitian, certified nutrition specialist, and master herbalist, Dr. Westerdahl diligently worked with me to explore ideas and challenge the norms to offer a comprehensive way to incorporate nutrition into the realm of health and beauty. His lifelong dedication to healthy eating is evident in the food menus he created within this book.

Dr. Westerdahl shared his years of experience as a former senior nutritionist for one of the leading international nutritional and herbal supplement companies. He is an American Dietetic Association panel member, serves on the faculty of the American Academy of Nutrition, and is a member of the American College of Nutrition. He is also the director of Wellness and Lifestyle Medicine for Castle Medical Center in Kailua, Hawaii, the nutrition editor for *Veggie Life* magazine, and a requested nutrition expert on many radio and television shows nationwide.

I am grateful and honored to have shared the experience of creating this book with both my son, Jeff, and Dr. Westerdahl.

Index

Page numbers in *italics* refer to illustrations and tables.